Surgical Approaches to the
Facial Skeleton

THIRD EDITION

Surgical Approaches to the

Facial Skeleton

THIRD EDITION

EDITORS

EDWARD ELLIS III, DDS, MS

Professor, Oral and Maxillofacial Surgery
Director of Residency Training
The University of Texas Southwestern Medical Center and
Chief of Oral and Maxillofacial Surgery
Parkland Memorial Hospital
Dallas, Texas

MICHAEL F. ZIDE, DMD

Associate Director, Oral and Maxillofacial Surgery
John Peter Smith Hospital
Fort Worth, Texas

VIDEO EDITORS

ERIC W. WANG, MD

Associate Professor
Department of Otolaryngology
University of Pittsburgh School of Medicine
Director
Maxillofacial Trauma
UPMC Presbyterian Hospital
Pittsburgh, Pennsylvania

JENNY Y. YU, MD

Vice Chair, Clinical Operations
Department of Ophthalmology
Assistant Professor
Department of Ophthalmology and Otolaryngology
University of Pittsburgh Medical Center
Pittsburgh, Pennsylvania

Illustrations by Jennifer Carmichael, MA and Lewis Calver, BFA, MS

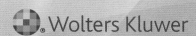

. Wolters Kluwer

Philadelphia · Baltimore · New York · London
Buenos Aires · Hong Kong · Sydney · Tokyo

Acquisitions Editor: Keith Donnellan
Marketing Manager: Stacy Malyil
Production Project Manager: Kim Cox
Design Coordinator: Stephen Druding
Editorial Coordinator: Dave Murphy
Manufacturing Coordinator: Beth Welsh
Prepress Vendor: SPi Global

Third edition

9 8 7 6 5 4 3 2 1

Printed in China

Library of Congress Cataloging-in-Publication Data
Names: Ellis, Edward, DDS, author. | Zide, Michael F., author.
Title: Surgical approaches to the facial skeleton / Edward Ellis, III, Michael F. Zide ; surgical videos by Eric W. Wang, Jenny Y. Yu.
Description: Third edition. | Philadelphia : Wolters Kluwer, [2018] | Includes bibliographical references and index.
Identifiers: LCCN 2017058293 | ISBN 9781496380418 (hardback)
Subjects: | MESH: Facial Bones—surgery
Classification: LCC RD523 | NLM WE 705 | DDC 617.5/2059—dc23 LC record available at https://lccn.loc.gov/2017058293

LWW.com

Plant a seed and it will grow.
There are many who have unknowingly contributed to this book through the education
they have provided me. All were my teachers, all are my friends. This book is dedicated
to these special individuals:

Robert Bruce

Amir El-Attar

W. James Gallo

James Hayward

Kazumas Kaya

Khursheed Moos

Timothy Pickens

Gilbert Small

George Upton

Al Weiss

EDWARD ELLIS III

In gratitude for ageless friendship and counsel. Doug Sinn, DDS, Jack Kent, DDS,
and Robert V. Walker, DDS.

To Riki: who puts up with me still.

MICHAEL F. ZIDE

PREFACE

There are many reasons for exposing the facial skeleton. Treatment of facial fractures, management of paranasal sinus disease, esthetic onlay and recontouring procedures, elective osteotomies, treatment of secondary traumatic deformities such as enophthalmos, placement of endosteal implants, and a host of other reconstructive procedures require approaches to the facial framework. Many approaches to a given skeletal region are possible. The choice is made usually on the basis of the surgeon's training, experience, and bias. This book does not advocate one approach over another, although the advantages and disadvantages of each approach will be listed. We maintain the age-old belief that "many roads lead to Rome." Therefore, the purpose of this book is to describe in detail the anatomical and technical aspects of most of the commonly used surgical approaches to the facial skeleton. We have deliberately not presented every approach, because many of them are not universally used, or are so simple that nothing needs to be said. However, the approaches presented in this book will allow the surgeon complete access to the craniofacial skeleton for whatever skeletal procedure is being performed.

We have attempted, from the beginning, to make Surgical Approaches to the Facial Skeleton different from the other books that touch on this subject. Most books that discuss surgical approaches do so in the context of the surgical procedure that is being presented. For instance, a book on facial fractures will usually present surgical approaches to a particular facial fracture. However, the surgical approach is not generally given much consideration or is it presented in sufficient detail for the novice. The reader is often left with the question, "How did the author get from the skin to that point on the skeleton?" We instead avoid consideration of why one is exposing the skeleton and describe the approaches in great detail so that even the novice can safely approach the facial skeleton by following the step-by-step description we have provided.

This book assumes that the reader has some basic understanding of regional anatomy, especially osteology. However, the anatomic structures of greatest interest will still be discussed for each surgical approach. This book also assumes that the reader has developed skills for the careful handling of soft tissues. We have suggested the use of those instruments that we have found useful for incising, retracting, and manipulating the tissues involved with each surgical approach, recognizing that others are also appropriate. The book also assumes that the reader is skilled in facial soft tissue closure. We have not discussed skin closure techniques associated with the approaches unless they differ from routine skin closures.

The first edition of Surgical Approaches to the Facial Skeleton became a hit with surgeons from several specialties when it was published in 1995. Oral and maxillofacial surgeons, plastic surgeons, and otolaryngologists all wanted this book for their collections. The book was most popular, however, among residents-in-training from these specialties.

The third edition of Surgical Approaches to the Facial Skeleton, like the first two editions, contains 14 chapters, 13 of which describe a specific surgical approach. The first chapter discusses basic principles involved in surgical approaches. The remaining 13 chapters are organized into sections, predominantly on the basis of the region of the face being exposed. There will often be more than one surgical approach presented for each region, with the choice left to the surgeon. We attempt to point out the advantages and disadvantages of each as they are presented.

The major change in the third edition of Surgical Approaches to the Facial Skeleton is the addition of videos. Drs. Eric Wang and Jenny Yu provide narrated videos that demonstrate 12 key approaches as performed on cadavers.

Edward Ellis III, DDS, MS
Michael F. Zide, DMD

CONTENTS

Preface   vii

Section 1   Basic Principles for Approaches to the Facial Skeleton   1

1   Basic Principles for Approaches to the Facial Skeleton 3

Section 2   Periorbital Incisions   7

2   Transcutaneous Approaches Through the Lower Eyelid 9
3   Transconjunctival Approaches. 41
4   Supraorbital Eyebrow Approach 65
5   Upper Eyelid Approach. 68

Section 3   Coronal Approach   79

6   Coronal Approach 81

Section 4   Transoral Approaches to the Facial Skeleton   109

7   Approaches to the Maxilla 111
8   Mandibular Vestibular Approach 137

Section 5   Transfacial Approaches to the Mandible   151

9   Submandibular Approach. 153
10   Retromandibular Approach 169
11   Rhytidectomy Approach 185

Section 6   Approaches to the Temporomandibular Joint   191

12   Preauricular Approach 193

Section 7	Surgical Approaches to the Nasal Skeleton	213

13 External (Open) Approach 215

14 Endonasal Approach 234

Index 247

Surgical Approaches to the
Facial Skeleton

THIRD EDITION

SECTION 1

Basic Principles for Approaches to the Facial Skeleton

1

Basic Principles for Approaches to the Facial Skeleton

Maximum success in skeletal surgery depends on adequate access to and exposure of the skeleton. Skeletal surgery is simplified and expedited when the involved parts are sufficiently exposed. In orthopaedic surgery, especially of the appendicular skeleton, the basic rule is to select the most *direct* approach possible to the underlying bone. Therefore, incisions are usually placed very near the area of interest while major nerves and blood vessels are retracted. This involves little regard for esthetics but allows the orthopaedic surgeon greater leeway in the location, direction, and length of the incision.

Surgery of the facial skeleton, however, differs from general orthopaedic surgery in several important ways. The first factor in incision placement is not surgical convenience but facial esthetics. The face is plainly visible to everyone, and a conspicuous scar may create a cosmetic deformity that can be as troubling to the individual as the reason for which the surgery was performed. Cosmetic considerations are critical in light of the emphasis that most societies place on facial appearance. Therefore, as we will see in this book, all the incisions made on the face must be placed in inconspicuous areas, sometimes distant from the underlying osseous skeleton on which the surgery is being performed. For instance, placement of incisions in the oral cavity allows superb exposure of most of the facial skeleton, with a completely hidden scar.

The second factor that differentiates incision placement on the face from incisions placed anywhere else on the body is the presence of the muscles and nerve (cranial nerve VII) of facial expression. The muscles are subcutaneous structures, and the branches of the facial nerve that supply them can be traumatized if incisions are made in their path. This can result in a "paralyzed" face, which is not only a severe cosmetic deformity but can also have great functional ramifications. For instance, if the ability to close the eye is lost, corneal damage can ensue, affecting vision. Therefore, placement of incisions and dissections that expose the facial skeleton must ensure that damage to the facial nerve is minimized. Many dissections to expose the skeleton require care and electrical nerve stimulation to identify and protect the nerve. Approaches using incisions in the facial skin must also take into consideration the muscles of facial expression. This is especially important for approaches to the orbit, where the orbicularis oculi muscle must be traversed. Closure of some incisions also affects the muscles of facial expression. For instance, if a maxillary vestibular incision is closed without proper reorientation of the perinasal muscles, the nasal base will widen.

The third factor in facial incision placement is the presence of many important sensory nerves exiting the skull at multiple locations. The facial soft tissues have more sensory input per unit area than soft tissues anywhere else in the body. Loss of this sensory input can be a great inconvenience to the individual. Therefore, the incisions and approaches used must avoid injury to the sensory nerves. An example is dissection of the supraorbital nerve from its foramen/notch in the coronal approach.

Other important factors are the patient's age, existing unique anatomy, and expectations. The age of the patient is important because of the possible presence of the wrinkles that come with age. Skin wrinkles serve as a guide and offer the surgeon the opportunity to place incisions within or parallel to them. Existing anatomic features that are unique to the individual can also facilitate or hamper incision placement. For instance, pre-existent lacerations can be used or extended to provide surgical exposure of the underlying skeleton. The position, direction, and depth of a laceration are important variables in determining its utility. The presence of old scars may also direct incision placement; the old scar may be excised and used to approach the skeleton. Sometimes, an old scar may not lend itself to use and may even cause the new incision to be positioned such that the old scar is avoided. Hair distribution may also direct the position of incisions. For instance, the incision for the coronal approach is largely determined by the patient's hairline. Ethnic characteristics also have a bearing on whether an incision will be placed in a conspicuous area. History or ethnic propensity for hypertrophic scarring, keloid formation, and hyper- or hypopigmentation may alter the decision as to whether or where to place an incision.

The patient's expectations and wishes must always be considered in any decision about location of an incision. For instance, patients who repeatedly require treatment of facial injuries may not be concerned with local cutaneous approaches to the naso-orbito-ethmoid region, whereas other individuals may be very concerned about the location of incisions. Therefore, the choice of surgical approach depends at least partly on the patient.

Principles of Incision Placement

Incisions placed in areas that are not readily visible, such as within the oral cavity or far behind the hairline, are not of esthetic concern. Incisions placed on exposed surfaces of the face, however, must follow some basic principles so that the scar will be less conspicuous. These principles are outlined in the following text.

Avoid Important Neurovascular Structures

Although this is an obvious consideration, avoiding anatomic hazards during placement of incisions is only a secondary consideration in the face. Instead, placing the incision in a cosmetically acceptable location takes priority. Important neurovascular structures encountered during the dissection must be dealt with by dissecting around them or by retracting them.

Use as Long an Incision as Necessary

Many surgeons tend to use short incisions. If the soft tissues around a short incision are stretched to obtain sufficient exposure of the skeleton, the additional trauma from retraction may create a less satisfactory scar than a longer incision would. A well-placed long incision may be less perceptible than a short incision that is placed poorly or requires great retraction. A long incision heals as quickly as a short one.

Place Incisions Perpendicular to the Surface of Non–hair-bearing Skin

Except in some very specific regions, an incision perpendicular to the skin surface permits the wound margins to be reapproximated in an accurate, layer-to-layer manner. Incisions performed obliquely to the surface of the skin are susceptible to marginal necrosis and to overlapping of the edges during closure. Incisions in hair-bearing tissue, however, should be parallel to the direction of the hair so that fewer follicles are transected. An oblique incision requires a more meticulous closure because of the tendency of the margins to overlap during suturing. Subcutaneous sutures may have to be placed more deeply to avoid necrosis of an oblique edge.

Place Incisions in the Lines of Minimal Tension

The lines of minimal tension, also called *relaxed skin tension lines*, are the result of the skin's adaptation to function and are also related to the elastic nature of the underlying dermis (see Fig. 1.1). The intermittent and chronic contractions of the muscles of facial expression create depressed creases in the skin of the face. These creases become more visible and depressed with age. For instance, the supraorbital wrinkle lines and the transverse lines of the forehead

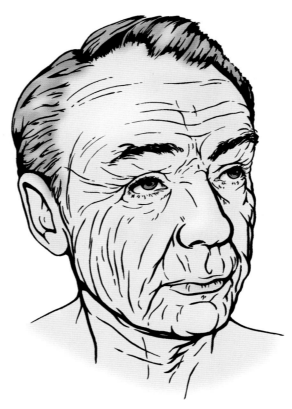

FIGURE 1.1 Lines of minimal tension (relaxed skin tension lines) are conspicuous in the aged face. These lines or creases are good choices for incision placement because the scars resulting from the incision will be imperceptible.

are caused by the contraction of the frontalis muscles, which insert into the skin of the lower forehead. In the upper eyelids, many fine perpendicular strands of fibers of the levator aponeurosis terminate in the dermis of the skin and along the tarsus to form the supratarsal fold. Similar insertions in the lower eyelid create fine horizontal lines, which are accentuated by the circumferential contraction of the orbicularis oculi muscle.

Incisions should be made within the lines of minimal tension. Incisions made within or parallel to such a line or crease will become inconspicuous if they are closed carefully. Any incision or portion of an incision that crosses such a crease, however, is often conspicuous.

Seek Other Favorable Sites for Incision Placement

If incisions cannot be placed within the lines of minimal tension, they can be made inconspicuous by placement inside an orifice, such as the mouth, nose, or eyelid; within hair-bearing areas or locations that can be covered by hair; or at the junction of two anatomic landmarks, such as the esthetic units of the face.

Periorbital Incisions

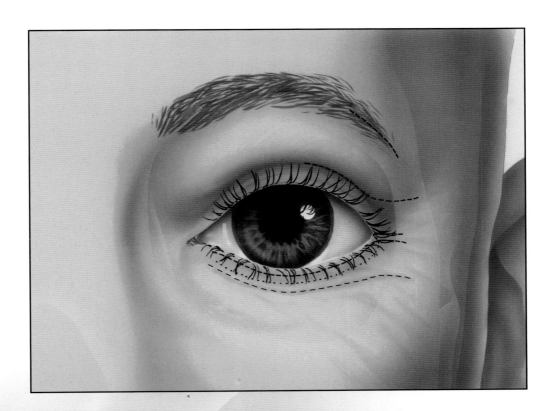

A standard series of incisions have been used extensively to approach the inferior, lateral, and medial orbital rims. Properly placed incisions offer excellent access with minimal morbidity and scarring. The most commonly used approaches are those made on the external surface of the lower eyelid, the conjunctival side of the lower eyelid, the skin of the lateral brow, and the skin of the upper eyelid. This section describes these approaches. Other periorbital approaches exist and can be useful. Existing lacerations of 2 cm or longer may also be used or extended to access the orbit.

2

Transcutaneous Approaches Through the Lower Eyelid

Approaches through the external side of the lower eyelid offer superb exposure to the inferior orbital rim, the floor of the orbit, the lateral orbit, and the inferior portion of the medial orbital rim and wall. These approaches are given many names in the literature (e.g., blepharoplasty, subciliary, lower- or mid-eyelid, subtarsal, infraorbital rim), based primarily on the position of the skin incision in the lower eyelid. Because of the natural skin creases in the lower eyelid and the thinness of eyelid skin, scars become inconspicuous with time and do not form keloids. The infraorbital incision, however, is almost always noticeable to some degree (see Fig. 2.1).

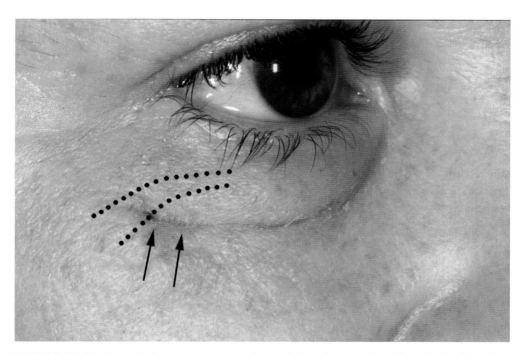

FIGURE 2.1 Photograph showing poor cosmetic result from the use of an infraorbital incision. Incisions placed at this level often heal poorly for two reasons: (a) the lateral extension of the incision usually crosses the resting skin tension lines (*dots*) that cause widening of the scar (*arrows*) and (b) the incision is in the thicker skin of the cheek rather than the thin skin of the eyelid.

Surgical Anatomy

Lower Eyelid

In the sagittal section, the lower eyelid (1) consists of at least four distinct layers: the skin and subcutaneous tissue, the orbicularis oculi muscle, the tarsus (upper 4 to 5 mm of the eyelid) or orbital septum, and the conjunctiva (see Fig. 2.2).

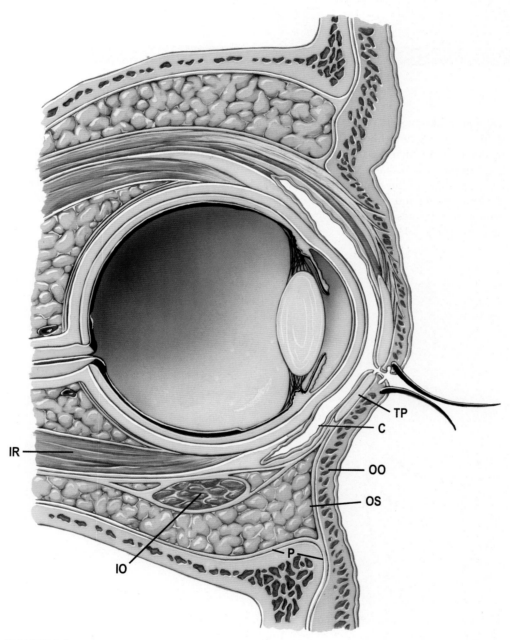

FIGURE 2.2 Sagittal section through the orbit and globe. *C*, palpebral conjunctiva; *IO*, inferior oblique muscle; *IR*, inferior rectus muscle; *OO*, orbicularis oculi muscle; *OS*, orbital septum; *P*, periosteum/periorbita; *TP*, tarsal plate.

Skin The skin is the outermost layer, and comprises the epidermis and the very thin dermis. The skin of the eyelids is the thinnest in the body and has many elastic fibers that allow it to be stretched during dissection and retraction. It is loosely attached to the underlying muscle; therefore, in contrast to most areas of the face, relatively large quantities of fluid may accumulate subcutaneously in this loose connective tissue. The skin derives its blood supply from the underlying perforating blood vessels of the muscles (see subsequent text).

Muscle The orbicularis oculi muscle, the sphincter of the eyelids, lies subjacent and adherent to the skin (see Fig. 2.3). This muscle completely encircles the palpebral fissure and extends over the skeleton of the orbit. It can therefore be divided into orbital and palpebral portions (see Fig. 2.4). The palpebral portion can be further subdivided into the pretarsal portion (i.e., the muscle superficial to the tarsal plates) and the preseptal portion (i.e., the muscle superficial to the orbital septum). The palpebral portion of the orbicularis oculi muscle is very thin in cross section, especially at the junction of the pretarsal and preseptal portions. The orbital portion of the orbicularis oculi muscle originates medially from the bones of the medial orbital rim and the medial canthal tendon. The peripheral fibers sweep across the eyelid over the orbital margin in a series of concentric loops, the more central ones forming almost complete rings. In the lower eyelid, the orbital portion extends below the inferior orbital rim onto the cheek and covers the origins of the elevator muscles of the upper lip and nasal ala. The orbital portion of the orbicularis oculi muscle is responsible for tight closure of the eye.

The preseptal portion of the orbicularis oculi muscle originates from the medial canthal tendon and lacrimal diaphragm and passes across the eyelid as a series of half-ellipses, meeting at the lateral canthal tendon. The upper and lower pretarsal muscles contribute to the lateral canthal tendon which extends approximately 7 mm before inserting lateral orbital tubercle. Medially, they unite to form the medial canthal tendon, which inserts on the medial orbital margin, the anterior lacrimal crest, and the nasal bones. The palpebral portion of the

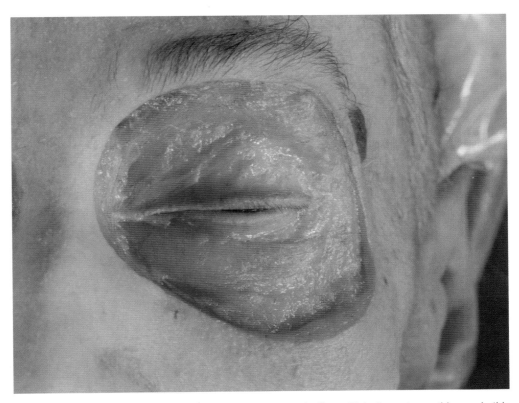

FIGURE 2.3 Anatomic dissection of orbicularis oculi muscle fibers. Note the extreme thinness in this older specimen.

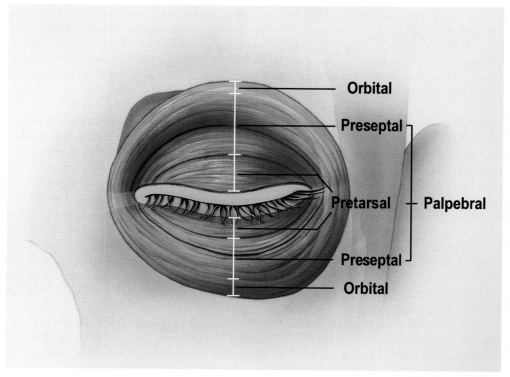

FIGURE 2.4 Orbital and palpebral portions of orbicularis oculi muscle. The palpebral portion is divided into the fibers in front of the tarsus (pretarsal portion) and those in front of the orbital septum (preseptal portion).

orbicularis oculi muscle functions to close the eye without effort, as in blinking. It also functions to maintain contact between the lower eyelid and the ocular globe.

The orbicularis oculi muscle is innervated laterally from the branches of the facial nerve that enter the muscle on its deeper surface. The blood supply to the orbicularis oculi muscle is from the external facial artery tributaries arising from the deep branches of the ophthalmic artery. These arterial branches form a marginal arcade, traversing between the tarsal plate and the muscle and giving rise to branches that perforate the substance of the muscle, the orbital septum, and the tarsal plate.

Orbital Septum/Tarsus The orbital septum is a fascial diaphragm between the contents of the orbit and the superficial face (Figs. 2.1 and 2.5). It is usually denser laterally than medially, but varies considerably in thickness from one individual to another, and weakens with age, allowing the orbital fat pads to bulge onto the face. The orbital septum is a fascial extension of the periosteum of the bones of the face and orbit. It originates along the orbital rim for most of its extent. Laterally and inferolaterally, however, it arises from the periosteum 1 to 2 mm beyond the rim of the orbit. Therefore, it is necessary to dissect a few millimeters lateral and/or inferior to the orbital rim before incising the periosteum to prevent incising through the orbital septum.

The orbital septum of the lower eyelid inserts into the inferior margin of the lower tarsus. The *tarsal plate* of the lower eyelid is a somewhat thin, pliable, fibrocartilaginous structure that gives form and support to the lower eyelid (see Fig. 2.6A and B). The edge of the tarsus that is adjacent to the free border of the eyelid is parallel to the palpebral fissure, whereas the deeper (inferior) border is curved such that the tarsus is somewhat semilunar in shape. It is also, of course, curved to conform to the outer surface of the eyeball. The inferior tarsus at approximately 4 to 5 mm is half the height of the superior tarsus (approximately 10 mm). The tarsal glands, sandwiched between the layers of fibrocartilage in the lower eyelid, are smaller than their upper eyelid counterpart, and exit on the eyelid margin

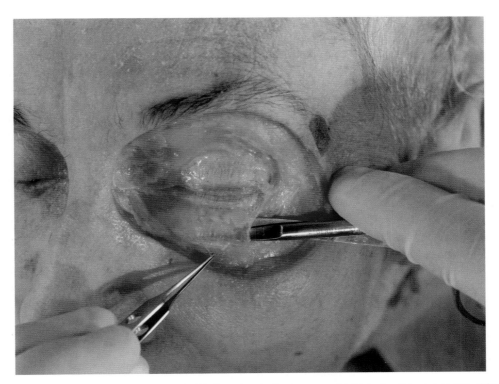

FIGURE 2.5 Anatomic dissection of orbital septum in the lower eyelid. Note the thinness in this older specimen.

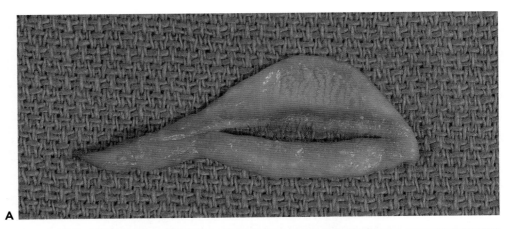

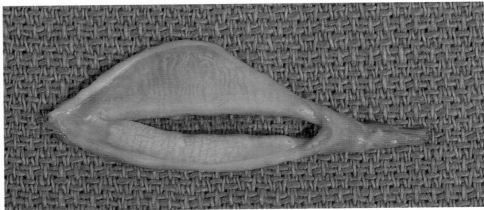

FIGURE 2.6 **A:** Anterior surface of tarsal plates and canthal tendons (left eye). Note the difference in size between the upper and lower tarsal plates. **B:** Posterior surface of the tarsal plates and canthal tendons (left eye). Note the vertically arranged Meibomian glands, visible through the thin conjunctiva.

near the lash follicles. The lashes are supported by their roots, which are attached to fibrous tissue on the tarsal plate and not in the orbicularis oculi muscle anterior to the tarsal plate. Laterally, the tarsal plate becomes a fibrous band that adjoins the structural counterpart from the upper eyelid, forming the lateral canthal tendon. Medially, the tarsal plate also becomes fibrous and shelters the inferior lacrimal canaliculus behind, as it becomes the medial canthal tendon.

Embedded within the tarsal plates are large sebaceous glands called the *tarsal* or *Meibomian glands*, whose ducts may be seen along the eyelid margin. A grayish line or a slight groove, which is sometimes visible between the lashes and the openings of the tarsal glands, represents the junction of the two fundamental portions of the eyelid: the skin and muscle on one hand and the tarsus (the plate of closely packed tarsal glands) and conjunctiva on the other. This junction indicates a plane along which the eyelid may be split into anterior and posterior portions with minimal scarring.

Palpebral Conjunctiva The conjunctiva that lines the inner surface of the eyelids is called the *palpebral conjunctiva* (Fig. 2.2). It adheres firmly to the tarsal plate, and as it extends inferiorly toward the inferior conjunctival fornix, it becomes more loosely bound. At the inferior conjunctival fornix, the conjunctiva sweeps onto the ocular globe to become the bulbar conjunctiva.

Lateral Canthal Tendon

The lateral canthal tendon, ligament, or *raphe* as it is frequently called, is a fibrous extension of the tarsal plates laterally toward the orbital rim (see Fig. 2.7). As will be seen in the medial canthal tendon, the lateral canthal tendon has a superficial and a deep component. The base of the ligamentous complex is "Y"-shaped and is attached to the external angle of the two

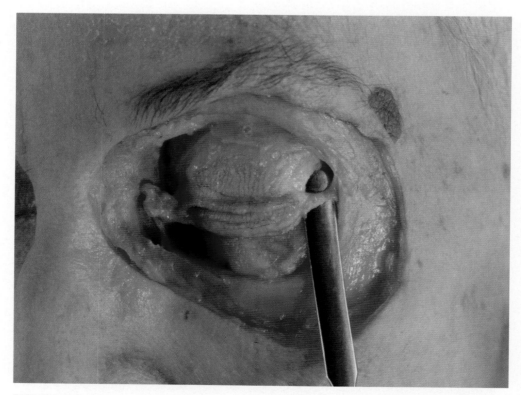

FIGURE 2.7 Anatomic dissection of the deep portion of the lateral canthal tendon. Note that it attaches posterior to the orbital rim.

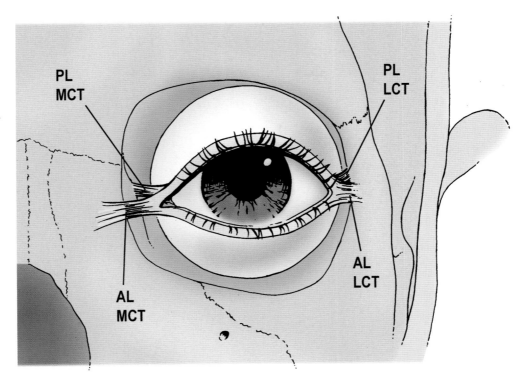

FIGURE 2.8 Medial and lateral canthal tendon complexes. Note that the anterior limb of the medial canthal tendon (*AL MCT*) and the posterior limb of the lateral canthal tendon (*PL LCT*) are thicker. The thick anterior portion of the medial canthal tendon attaches to the anterior lacrimal crest of the maxilla and the frontal process of the maxilla. The thinner *PL MCT* attaches along the posterior lacrimal crest of the lacrimal bone. The thick *PL LCT* attaches to the orbital (Whitnall) tubercle of the zygoma, 3 to 4 mm posterior to the lateral orbital rim. The thinner anterior fibers course laterally to mingle with the orbicularis oculi muscle fibers and the periosteum of the lateral orbital rim.

tarsi (see Fig. 2.8). The two divisions diverge from the tarsi and the superficial component extends laterally just under, or intermingles with, the orbicularis oculi muscle. It continues laterally to the orbital rim and inserts into the periosteum overlying the lateral orbital rim and the temporalis fascia just lateral to the orbital rim. The superficial limb coalesces with the temporal periosteum over the lateral orbital rim. The thicker, stronger deep component of the lateral canthal tendon courses posterolaterally, inserting into the periosteum of the orbital tubercle of the zygoma, approximately 3 to 4 mm posterior to the orbital rim. The space between the two bundles of the lateral canthal tendon is filled with loose connective tissue.

Medial Canthal Tendon

The medial canthal tendon is attached to the medial bony orbit by the superficial and the deep components that attach to the anterior and posterior lacrimal crests (see Figs. 2.8 and 2.9) (2,3). The medial canthal tendon originates at the nasal border of the upper and lower tarsi, where the preseptal muscles divide into superficial and deep heads (4). The lacrimal puncta are located here. Therefore, the lacrimal canaliculi of the upper and lower eyelid margins extend from the medial border of the tarsi toward and behind the medial canthus. Continuing medially, the tendon fans out to insert into the anterior lacrimal crest and beyond onto the frontal process of the maxilla. The anterior lacrimal crest, which is 2 to 3 mm medial to the canthal apex, protects the lacrimal sac. Therefore, an incision farther medial than 3 mm from the canthus misses both the canaliculi and the sac.

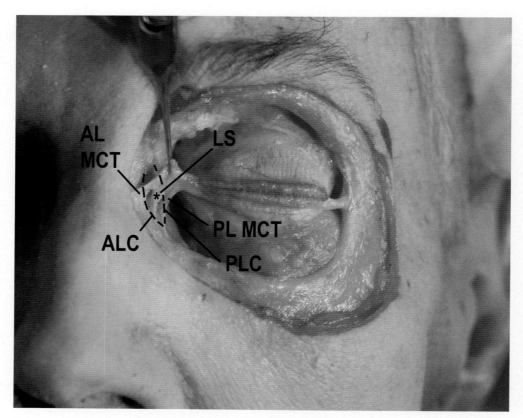

FIGURE 2.9 Anatomic specimen showing the anterior and posterior components of the medial canthal tendon complex. *AL MCT*, anterior limb of the medial canthal tendon; *ALC*, anterior lacrimal crest; *LS*, lacrimal sac; *PL MCT*, posterior limb of the medial canthal tendon; *PLC*, posterior lacrimal crest.

The anterior horizontal segment is the strongest component of the medial canthal tendon complex and is attached most firmly at the anterior lacrimal crest. The thinner posterior limb inserts into the posterior lacrimal crest and functions to maintain the eyelids in a posture tangential to the globe. The resultant vector of all the canthal attachments suggests that resuspension of the entire complex following disruption should be posterior and superior to the anterior lacrimal crest.

Infraorbital Groove

The infraorbital neurovascular bundle enters the posterior orbit through the inferior orbital fissure and runs almost straight anteriorly in the infraorbital groove of the orbital floor (see Fig. 2.10). More anteriorly, the infraorbital groove is usually covered with a thin layer of bone, forming the infraorbital canal, which leads the neurovascular bundle through the infraorbital foramen to the superficial structures of the face. The superior alveolar nerves split off the infraorbital nerve at a depth of 5 to 25 mm within the infraorbital canal and give sensation to the maxillary teeth and gingiva.

Techniques

Several external incisions of the lower eyelid to allow access to the infraorbital rim and orbital floor have been described. The major difference between these incisions is the level at which they are placed on the skin of the eyelid and the level at which the muscle is transected to expose the orbital septum/periosteum. Each incision has advantages and disadvantages.

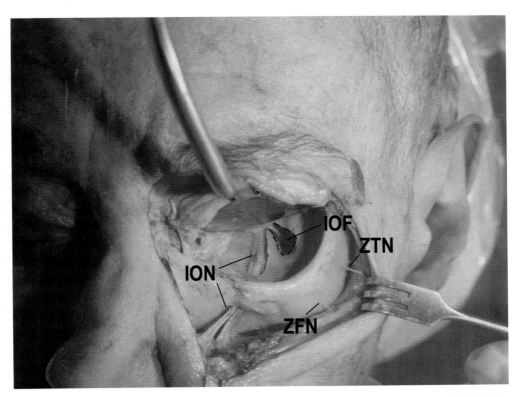

FIGURE 2.10 Anatomic dissection of the orbital floor, lateral and inferior orbital rims. *IOF*, inferior orbital fissure after incision of contents; *ION*, infraorbital nerve in canal/groove after unroofing; *ZFN*, zygomaticofacial nerve; *ZTN*, zygomaticotemporal nerve.

The two approaches and one modification are illustrated in the following text. The first is most commonly called the *subciliary incision*, also known as the *infraciliary* or *blepharoplasty incision*. This incision is made just below the eyelashes. The advantages of this incision are the imperceptible scar and the ease of extending laterally for additional exposure of the entire lateral orbital rim. The second approach is usually known as the *subtarsal*, also known as the *mid-eyelid* or *skin crease approach*, because the incision is made lower than that in the subciliary approach, often 4 to 7 mm below the eyelid margin. The subciliary approach will be shown in great detail. The subtarsal approach will be contrasted to the subciliary approach. In addition to these approaches, a modification of the subciliary approach, which can provide access to the entire lateral rim and internal wall of the orbit, will also be illustrated.

Technique for Subciliary Approach

The skin incision is made just below the eyelashes. Three surgical paths are available to access the orbital rim—the "skin flap" dissection, the "skin–muscle" flap dissection, and the "step" dissection. Briefly, the "skin flap" approach involves dissecting the thin eyelid skin from the subciliary incision down to the level of the orbital rim. Subsequently, the orbicularis oculi and the periosteum are transected just below the orbital rim. The "skin–muscle" flap proceeds through both the skin and the pretarsal muscle, directly atop the inferior tarsal plate, and dissects down the orbital septum, toward the orbital rim, where an incision is made through the periosteum to the bone. The "step" dissection is technically easier and abrogates the common complications associated with the other two methods, namely, skin or septal buttonholes, darkening of the skin, ectropion, and occasionally entropion.

The "step" dissection preserves pretarsal fibers of the orbicularis oculi, thereby limiting scarring at the eyelid margin and maintaining the position of the eyelid and its contact with the globe (Video 2.1).

➤ **STEP 1.** Protection of the Globe

Protecting the cornea during surgical procedures around the orbit may reduce ocular injuries. If surgery is performed on the skin side of the eyelids to approach the orbital rim and/or orbital floor, a temporary tarsorrhaphy or scleral shell may be useful. These are simply removed on completion of the surgery (see Figs. 2.11 and 2.12).

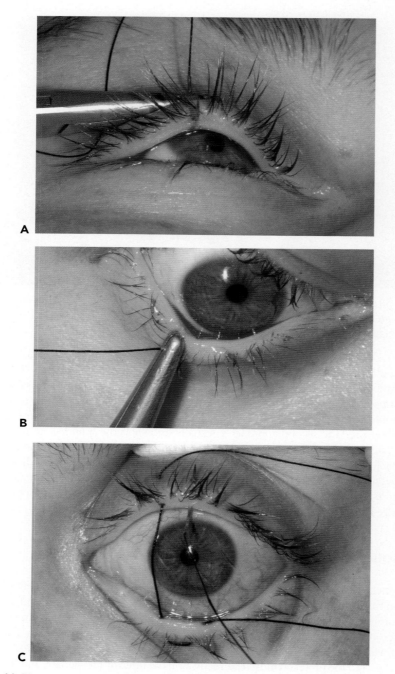

FIGURE 2.11 Placement of tarsorrhaphy suture. **A:** A 4-0 silk suture is passed through the skin of the upper eyelid and is directed through the *gray line* of the upper lid margin. Two methods can be used for placing the tarsorrhaphy suture through the lower eyelid. **B:** The suture is passed into and out of the *gray line* in a single pass without exiting the skin. The suture should be passed deep enough to get a good bite of the inferior tarsus to prevent it from being pulled out. **C** and **D:** An alternative method using a horizontal mattress suture in which the needle is passed from the superior portion of the lower eyelid (*gray line*) out of the skin, and back again. The final pass of the suture is through the *gray line* of the upper eyelid, exiting the skin. Either technique works well.

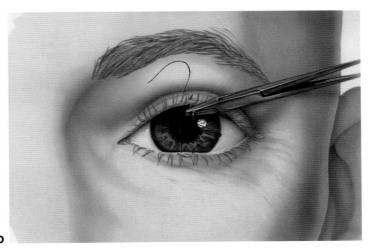

FIGURE 2.11 (*continued*)

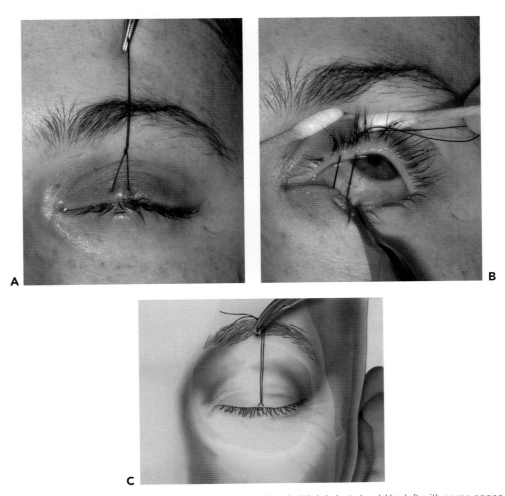

FIGURE 2.12 A: The tarsorrhaphy suture should not be tied tightly but should be left with some space between the knot and the skin of the upper eyelid because it may be necessary to open the palpebral fissure slightly during the surgery to examine the eye and/or to perform forced duction tests **(B)**. **C:** A hemostat can be used to grasp the tarsorrhaphy suture to apply traction to the lower eyelid during incision and dissection.

➤   **STEP 2.** Identification and Marking of the Incision Line

The incision for a subciliary approach is made approximately 2 mm inferior to the lashes, along the entire length of the eyelid (see Fig. 2.13A). The incision may be extended laterally approximately 2 cm past the lateral canthus without damaging the anterior temporal branch of the facial nerve (which crosses the zygomatic arch at 3 cm from the canthus) preferably in a natural crease. If a natural skin crease is not obvious, the extension can usually be made straight laterally or slightly inferolaterally.

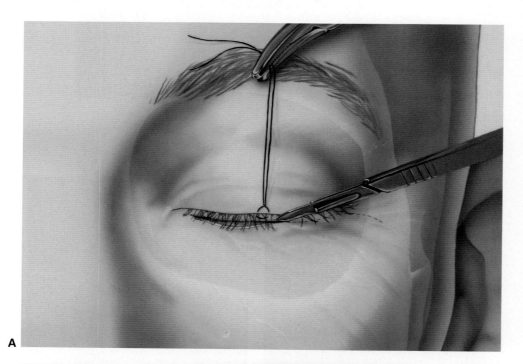

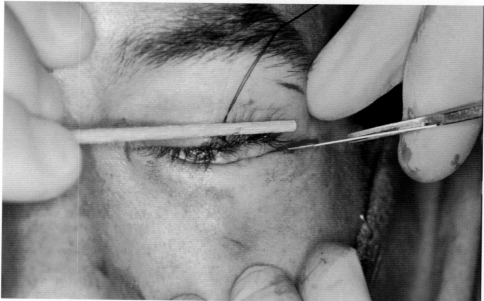

FIGURE 2.13 Subciliary incision being made. **A:** The incision is approximately 2 mm below the eyelashes and can be extended laterally as necessary (*top dashed line*). It is made through skin *only*. **B:** A Freer elevator or a cotton-tipped applicator stick can be used to lift the lower eyelashes to prevent them from being injured during the incision.

➤ **STEP 3.** Vasoconstriction

Ideally, the incision line is inked *before* infiltration of a vasoconstrictor. Tissues distort after infiltration and a perceptible crease may disappear following the injection. If the eyelid is swollen and creases are effaced, consider an injection of hyaluronidase (150 U) mixed in 30 mL of local anesthesia with a vasoconstrictor. Dilute epinephrine solutions not only aid in hemostasis but can also separate the tissue planes before the incision, thereby facilitating incision in the thin eyelids.

➤ **STEP 4.** Skin Incision

The depth of the initial incision is through the skin *only*. The underlying muscle should be visible when the skin is incised completely (Fig. 2.13A and B).

➤ **STEP 5.** Subcutaneous Dissection

Subcutaneous dissection toward the inferior orbital rim proceeds for a few millimeters using sharp dissection with a scalpel or scissors. The tissue should be tented "up" rather than pulled "back" to avoid dehiscence (see Figs. 2.14 and 2.15). The tarsorrhaphy suture is used to retract the lower eyelid superiorly to assist in the dissection. The skin should be separated from the pretarsal portion of the orbicularis oculi muscle along the entire extent of the incision. Approximately 4 to 6 mm of subcutaneous dissection is adequate.

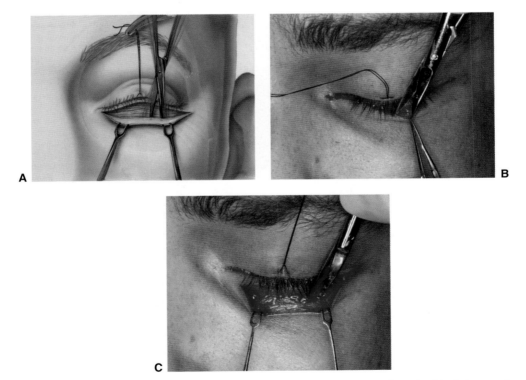

FIGURE 2.14 A: Subcutaneous dissection of skin, leaving pretarsal portion of orbicularis muscle attached to the tarsus. **B** and **C:** Dissection 4 to 6 mm inferiorly in this plane is adequate.

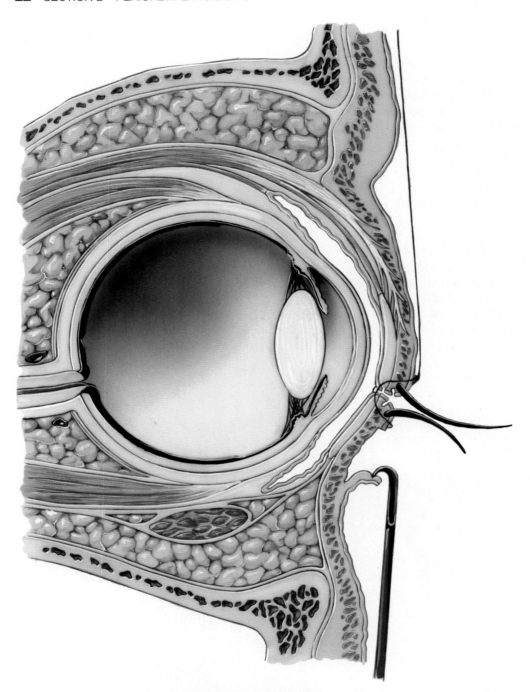

FIGURE 2.15 Sagittal plane through the orbit and globe demonstrating the subcutaneous dissection of the lid margin.

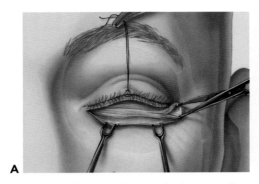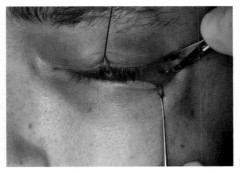

A **B**

FIGURE 2.16 A and **B:** Use of scissors to dissect through orbicularis oculi muscle over lateral orbital rim to identify periosteum.

➤ **STEP 6.** Suborbicularis Dissection

Scissors with slightly blunted tips are used to dissect through the orbicularis oculi muscle (by spreading in the direction of the muscle) to the periosteum overlying the lateral orbital rim (see Fig. 2.16A and B). Initially, the muscle is dissected over the bony rim because this area is *always* anterior to the septum orbitale. Limited supraperiosteal dissection in this submuscular plane, over the anterior edge of the infraorbital rim, produces a perfect pocket to cleanly dissect superficial to the septum orbitale. Scissors are used to spread upward in this pocket into the lower eyelid, with the upper tine of the scissors directly beneath the "step" incision and the lower tine over the orbital rim (see Figs. 2.17 and 2.18). In this plane between the orbicularis oculi muscle and the orbital septum, the convexity of the curved scissors faces outward.

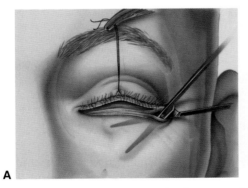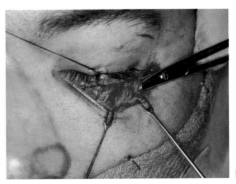

A **B**

FIGURE 2.17 A and **B:** Dissection between orbicularis oculi muscle and orbital septum. The dissection should extend completely along the orbital rim and superiorly to the level of subcutaneous dissection.

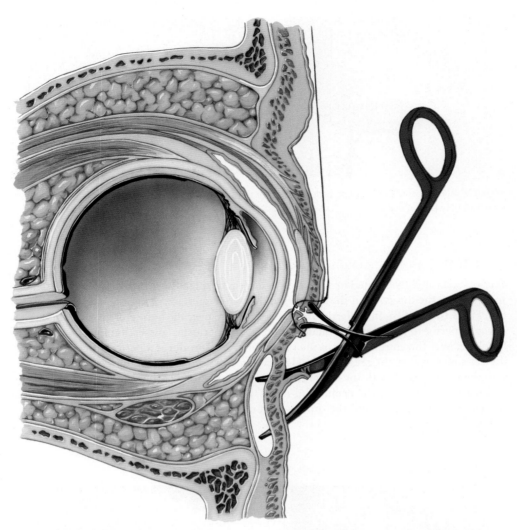

FIGURE 2.18 Sagittal plane through orbit showing the level and extent of dissection. Note the bridge of orbicularis oculi muscle remaining between the lid and skin–muscle flap.

➤ **STEP 7.** Incision Between Pretarsal and Preseptal Portions of Orbicularis Oculi Muscle

An attachment of the orbicularis oculi muscle will remain, extending from the tarsal plate to the skin–muscle flap, which was just elevated from the orbital septum (see Fig. 2.19). This muscle is now incised with scissors placed inferior to the level of the initial skin incision (see Fig. 2.20).

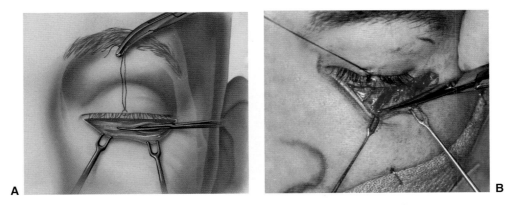

FIGURE 2.19 **A** and **B:** Incision through the bridge of the orbicularis oculi muscle.

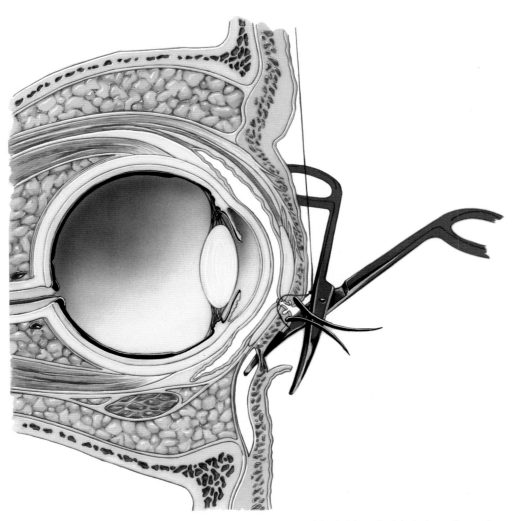

FIGURE 2.20 Sagittal plane through orbit showing incision of the bridge of orbicularis oculi muscle.

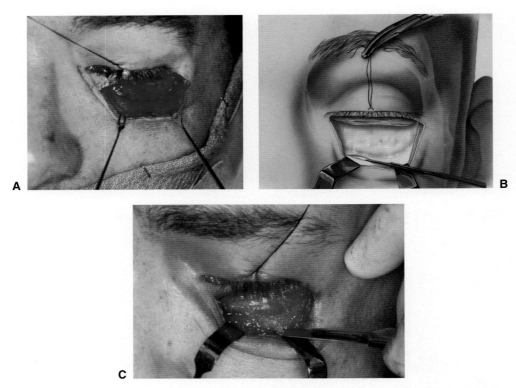

FIGURE 2.21 A: Photograph showing retraction of the flap in preparation for periosteal incision. Note that the orbital septum is intact. **B:** Incision through periosteum along anterior maxilla, 3 to 4 mm inferior to infraorbital rim. Note that the pretarsal muscle is still remaining on the inferior tarsus and the orbital septum, which restricts the orbital fat from entering the field **(C)**.

> ### STEP 8. Periosteal Incision

Once the skin–muscle flap of tissue is elevated from the lower eyelid, it can be retracted inferiorly, extending below the inferior orbital rim (see Fig. 2.21A). If the orbital septum is not violated, the tarsal plate above it should be visible with the pretarsal portion of orbicularis oculi still attached and with the orbital septum below extending to the infraorbital rim. An incision can be made with a scalpel through the periosteum on the *anterior* surface of the maxilla and zygoma, 3 to 4 mm below or lateral to the orbital rim (Fig. 2.21B and C). The incision through the periosteum at this level avoids the insertion of the orbital septum along the orbital margin. The infraorbital nerve is approximately 5 to 7 mm inferior to the orbital rim and should be avoided when the periosteal incision is made.

> ### STEP 9. Subperiosteal Dissection of Anterior Maxilla and/or Orbit

The sharp end of a periosteal elevator is pulled across the full length of the periosteal incision to separate the incised edges. Periosteal elevators are then used to strip the periosteum from the underlying osseous skeleton, both along the anterior surface of the maxilla and zygoma and inside the orbit. The inferior orbital rim is superior to the orbital floor just behind it. After the periosteum of the infraorbital rim is elevated (see Fig. 2.22A), the elevator is positioned vertically, stripping inferiorly as it proceeds posteriorly for the first centimeter or so (Fig. 2.22A–D). The bony origin of the inferior oblique muscle (the only muscle in the orbit that does not arise from its apex) will be stripped during the subperiosteal dissection.

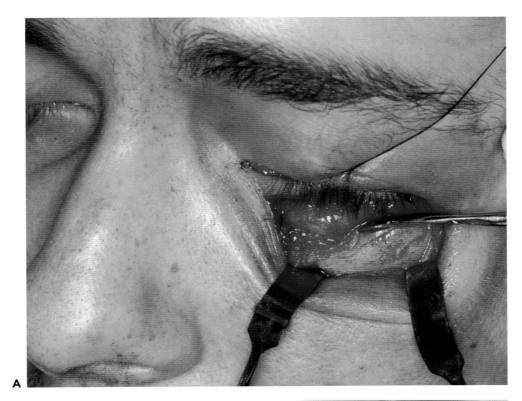

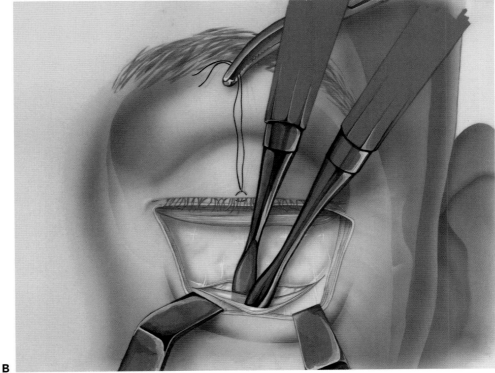

FIGURE 2.22 A: Photograph showing elevation of periosteum over the top of the infraorbital rim. Frontal **(B)** and sagittal **(C)** illustrations showing subperiosteal dissection of anterior maxilla and orbital floor. Note that the periosteal elevator entering the orbit is placed almost vertically **(D)** as dissection proceeds behind the rim. In the anterior region, the floor of the orbit is at a lower level than the crest of the rim, necessitating dissection inferiorly just behind the crest of the rim.

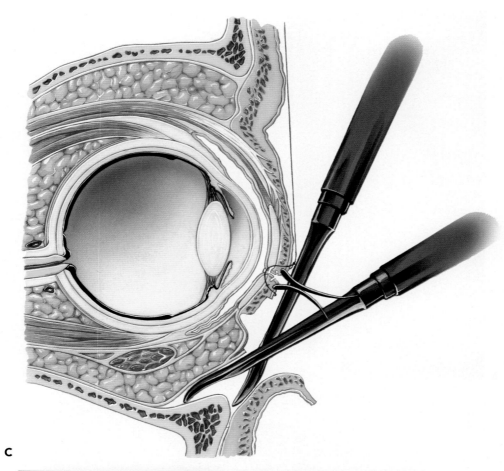

C

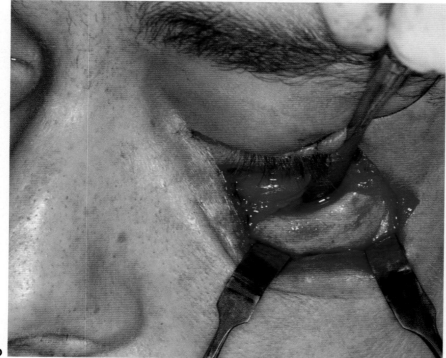

D

FIGURE 2.22 *(continued)*

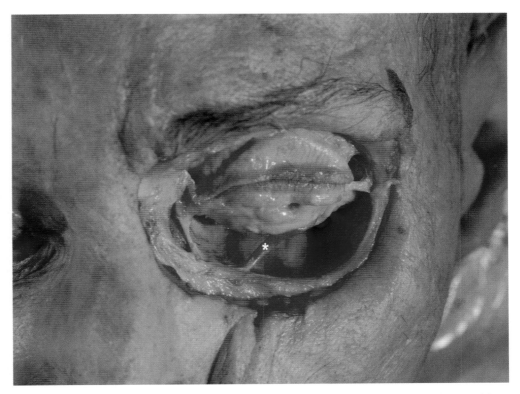

FIGURE 2.23 Anatomic dissection showing the position of the inferior oblique muscle (*). It should not be directly visualized if one stays in the subperiosteal plane because its origin will be stripped from the orbital floor along with the periosteum.

The muscle arises from the floor of the medial orbit just posterior to the orbital rim and lateral to the upper aperture of the nasolacrimal canal and may also arise partly from the lacrimal fascia over the lacrimal sac (see Fig. 2.23). During dissection, one will readily encounter the inferior orbital fissure. The periosteum of the orbit (periorbita) sweeps downward into the fissure. When indicated for exposure, the contents of the inferior orbital fissure may be safely incised after bipolar cautery (see Fig. 2.24A and B). Superior retraction of the orbital contents exposes the orbital floor and walls, as well as the anterior maxilla (see Fig. 2.25).

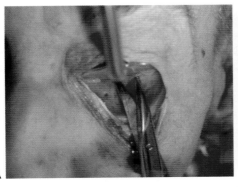
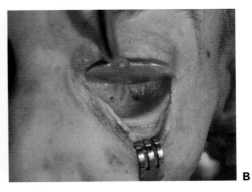

FIGURE 2.24 A: Anatomic dissection showing incision through the contents of the inferior orbital fissure to facilitate orbital dissection. These tissues should first be cauterized with bipolar electrocoagulation to prevent bleeding when incised. **B:** Anatomic dissection showing increased exposure of the orbit after incision of contents of the inferior orbital fissure.

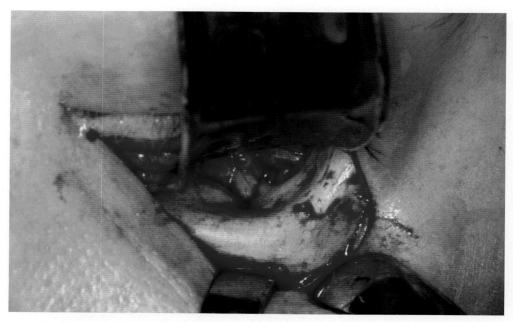

FIGURE 2.25 Photograph showing the internal orbit after dissection.

➤ **STEP 10.** Closure

Closure is usually performed in two layers: the periosteum and the skin (see Fig. 2.26A). Periosteal resorbable sutures ensure that the soft tissues stripped from the anterior surface of the maxilla and zygoma are repositioned anatomically (Fig. 2.26B). Suturing of the orbicularis oculi muscle is unnecessary unless it has been cut vertically or stripped excessively over the zygomatic prominence. Resorbable sutures may be inserted laterally, where the incised orbicularis oculi muscle is thicker (see Fig. 2.27).

A 6-0 nonresorbable or fast-resorbing suture is then run along the skin margin.

➤ **STEP 11.** Suspensory Suture for Lower Eyelid

Any incision or laceration used to gain access to the infraorbital rim and orbital floor may shorten the lower eyelid vertically during healing. Skin and septal scarring may be beneficially counteracted by superior support of the lower eyelid for several days (or until gross edema has resolved) after surgery. The simplest method is to run a suture through the gray line of the lower eyelid, which is taped to the forehead (see Fig. 2.28). This lifts and supports the lower eyelid in a lengthened position while eyelid edema dissipates.

To eliminate suture slippage during functional postoperative forehead motion, a first layer of tape is applied to the skin. The suture is positioned over the first layer and a second tape is applied over it. The suture is folded over this second tape and a third strip of tape is applied over the suture and the other two strips.

Vision may be checked by opening the upper eyelid. The entire anterior surface of the globe can be examined by simply removing the tape from the forehead and opening both eyelids.

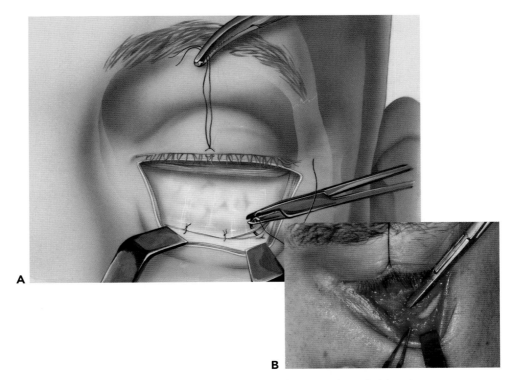

FIGURE 2.26 **A** and **B:** Closure of the periosteum with interrupted resorbable sutures.

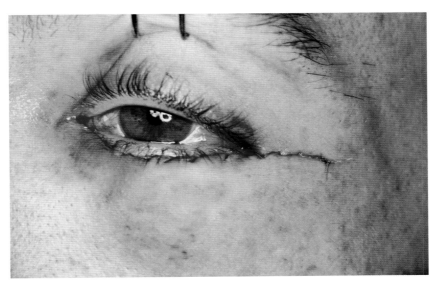

FIGURE 2.27 Photograph showing closure with running 6-0 nonresorbable suture.

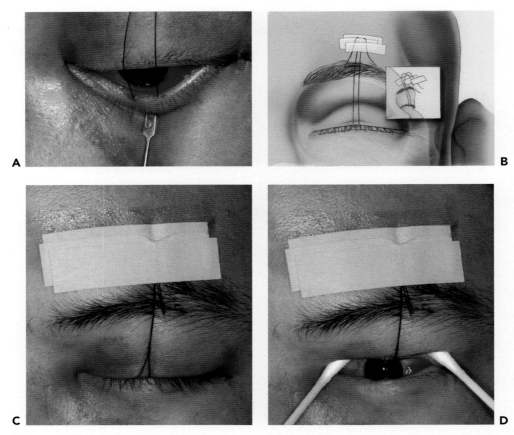

FIGURE 2.28 Lower-eyelid suspensory suture placed at completion of surgery. The suture is placed through the *gray line* of the lower eyelid, into the tarsus, and then exits the *gray line* at approximately 5 mm from the point where it entered **(A)**. It is important to engage some of the tarsal plate to prevent the suture from being pulled out. It is taped to the forehead in the manner shown to provide firm suspension **(B and C)**. The suspension suture does not engage the upper eyelid, leaving it free to permit examination of the eye **(D)**.

Technique for Subtarsal Approach

The technique for the subtarsal approach has many of the same maneuvers as that described for the subciliary approach, such as protection of the globe, vasoconstriction, and dissection of the orbit. Only those salient points that are different from the ones just described for the subciliary approach are presented here (Video 2.2).

Identification and Marking of the Incision Line

The skin incision for the subtarsal approach is approximately at the level of the inferior margin of the lower tarsus, in the subtarsal fold. In practice, however, it is made in a natural skin crease in the middle of the lower eyelid (see Fig. 2.29). Although the final scar in this location may be slightly more perceptible than the subciliary incision, clinical investigations reveal a lower incidence of scleral show and ectropion with this approach (5,6).

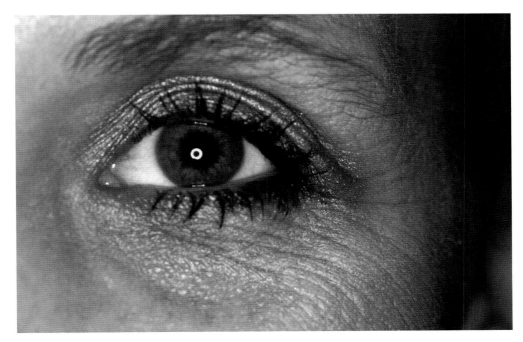

FIGURE 2.29 Photograph showing resting skin tension lines around the eyelids. Any one of these tension lines can be chosen for incision placement, or an incision can be made parallel to them.

The skin creases around the orbit should be evaluated carefully (see Fig. 2.30A). If the tissue is swollen, the skin of the opposite orbit may be used to assess and to appreciate the direction of creases. Usually, the crease tails off inferiorly as it extends laterally (Fig. 2.29). If access to the orbital floor and inferior orbital rim are all that is necessary, the subtarsal incision is satisfactory and will result in an imperceptible scar. Extension of the mid-eyelid incision follows the natural crease and never deviates superiorly toward the eyelid margin.

The incision line is marked *before* infiltration of a vasoconstrictor (Fig. 2.30B).

Skin Incision

The initial incision is through skin and muscle, to the depth of the orbital septum (Fig. 2.30C and D). The incision extends laterally just past the bone of the lateral orbital rim. The skin–muscle flap is then elevated from the orbital septum as dissection proceeds inferiorly. Any remaining orbicularis muscle is dissected at the level of the orbital septum with scissors in a spreading motion and is then incised (Fig. 2.30E and F).

Suborbicularis Dissection

Scissors with slightly blunted tips are used to dissect between the orbicularis oculi muscle and the orbital septum (Fig. 2.30G and H). A double skin-hook is used to retract the incised lower eyelid skin–muscle flap, and dissection proceeds in this submuscular plane inferiorly along the lateral rim, over the anterior edge of the infraorbital rim (Fig. 2.30I).

The incision through the periosteum (Fig. 2.30J and K), the dissection of the orbit (Fig. 2.30L), and closure (Fig. 2.30M–Q) are the same as described for the subciliary approach.

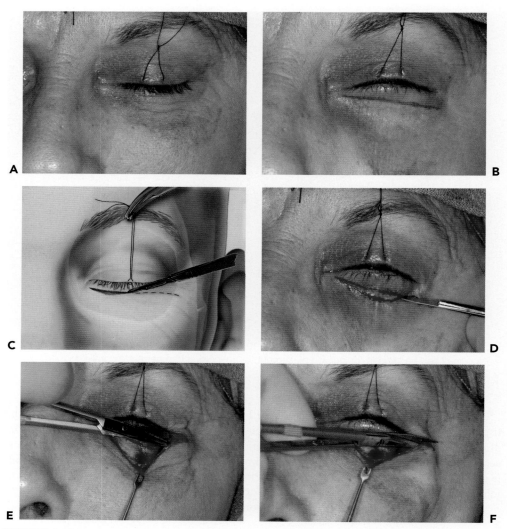

FIGURE 2.30 Subtarsal approach to the orbit. **A:** Photograph prior to incision demonstrating the natural eyelid creases for this patient. **B:** Incision marked. **C:** Illustration and **(D)** photograph showing the incision being made. **E:** Scissors dissecting orbicularis oculi muscle laterally along the orbital rim, just superficial to the orbital septum. **F:** Scissors incising the orbicularis oculi muscle. **G:** Illustration showing the level of dissection. **H:** Scissors dissecting inferiorly toward the infraorbital rim. **I:** Appearance after the skin–muscle flap has been elevated to the infraorbital rim (*S*, orbital septum; *OO*, orbicularis oculi muscle). **J:** Illustration showing elevation of the skin–muscle flap and incision through the periosteum along the anterior maxilla just below the orbital rim. **K:** Incision through the periosteum being made with electrocautery. **L:** Dissection into the orbit. **M:** Resorbable suture being passed through the periosteum on both sides of the incision. **N:** Appearance after periosteal closure. **O:** Resorbable suture (knot buried) passed through orbicularis oculi muscle on each side of incision. **P:** Appearance after orbicularis oculi muscle sutures placed. **Q:** Final closure with running 6-0 fast absorbing catgut suture.

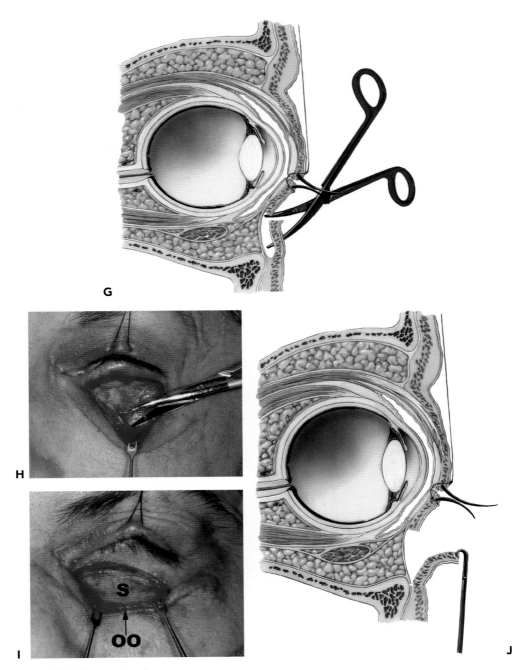

FIGURE 2.30 *(continued)*

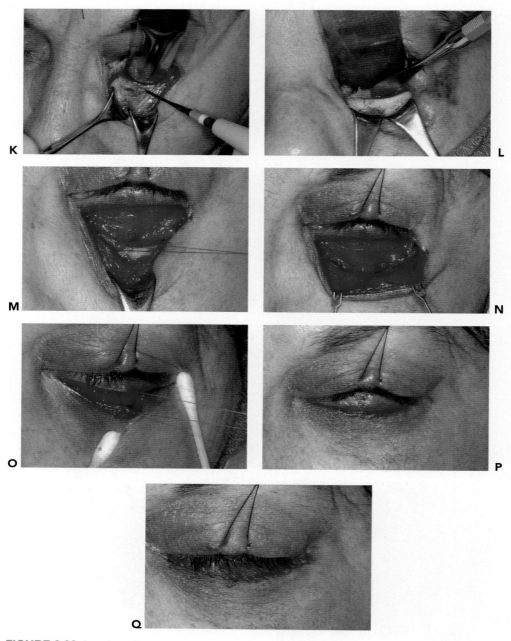

FIGURE 2.30 *(continued)*

Alternative Technique: Extended Lower Eyelid Approach

The extended lower eyelid approach provides access to the entire lateral orbital rim to a point approximately 10 to 12 mm superior to the frontozygomatic suture (7). Although less direct, this access may substitute for the lateral brow or upper eyelid approaches. For unrestricted exposure, the lateral canthal tendon must be stripped from its insertions and subsequently repositioned. This approach is useful when the entire lateral orbit, lateral orbital rim, orbital floor, and inferior orbital rim have to be accessed.

The incision for the *extended* subciliary approach is exactly the same as that described for the standard subciliary incision, but the incision must be extended laterally by approximately 1 to 1.5 cm in a natural crease (Fig. 2.13). If no natural skin crease extends laterally from the lateral palpebral fissure, the extension can usually be made straight laterally, or slightly infero-laterally. The subtarsal approach does not lend itself to this extended dissection because the incision is placed more inferiorly than the subciliary incision, especially laterally where the dissection up the lateral orbital rim proceeds.

Supraperiosteal dissection of the entire lateral orbital rim is performed with scissors dissection to a point above the frontozygomatic suture (see Fig. 2.31). The orbicularis oculi musculature and the superficial portion of the lateral canthal tendon are retracted superiorly.

The periosteum is then incised in the middle of the lateral orbital rim from the superior extent downwards, connecting to the standard infraorbital rim incision (see Fig. 2.32). Subperiosteal dissection strips the tissues from the orbital floor and lateral orbital wall, including insertions of the deep component of the lateral canthal tendon, Lockwood suspensory ligament, and the lateral check ligament from the orbital (Whitnall) tubercle of the zygoma. The frontozygomatic suture is readily exposed (see Fig. 2.33).

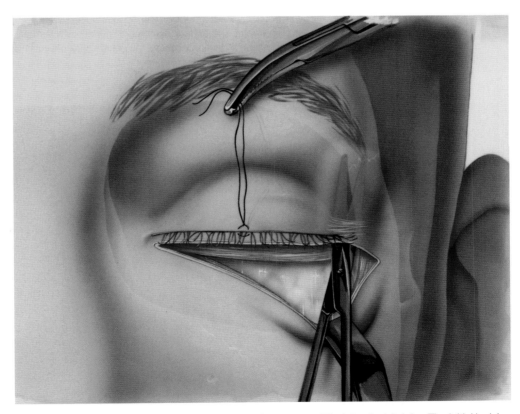

FIGURE 2.31 Technique used to obtain increased exposure of the lateral orbital rim. The initial incision is extended laterally 1 to 1.5 cm, and supraperiosteal dissection along the lateral orbital rim proceeds superiorly until the area of interest is approached.

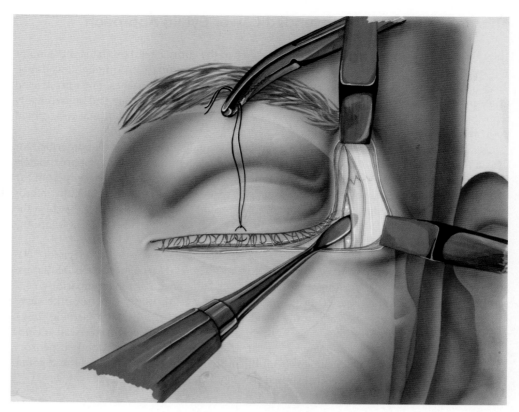

FIGURE 2.32 Dissection to the level of the frontozygomatic suture. The tissues superficial to the periosteum are retracted superiorly with a small retractor and an incision through periosteum is made 3 to 4 mm lateral to the lateral orbital rim. Subperiosteal dissection exposes the entire lateral orbital rim. Dissection into the lateral orbit frees the tissues and allows retraction superiorly.

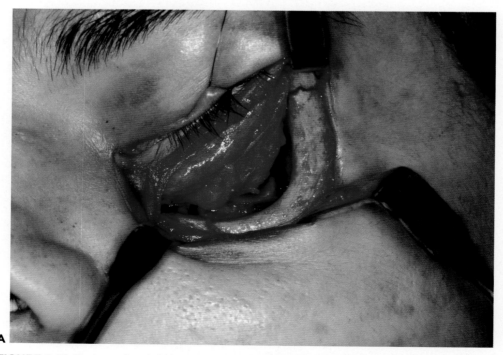

FIGURE 2.33 Photographs after "extended" subciliary approach. **A:** Entire lateral orbital rim exposed to a level above the frontozygomatic suture. **B:** Orbital floor exposure (fractured). **C:** Lateral orbital wall (greater wing of sphenoid and zygoma) exposed.

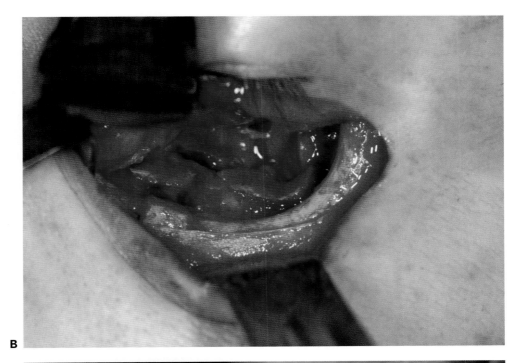

B

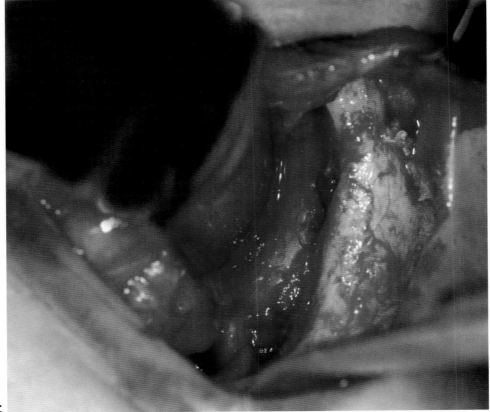

C

FIGURE 2.33 *(continued)*

Isolated lateral canthopexy is not necessary if careful repositioning and suturing of the periosteum along the lateral orbital rim are accomplished. This maneuver brings the superficial portion of the lateral canthal tendon into proper position, giving the lateral palpebral fissure a satisfactory appearance.

REFERENCES

1. Zide BM, Jelks GW. *Surgical anatomy of the orbit*. New York: Raven Press; 1985.
2. Anderson RC. The medial canthal tendon branches out. *Arch Ophthalmol*. 1977;95:2051.
3. Zide BM, McCarthy JG. The medial canthus revisited. An anatomical basis for canthopexy. *Ann Plast Surg*. 1983;11:1.
4. Rodriguez RL, Zide BM. Reconstruction of the medial canthus. *Clin Plast Surg*. 1988;15:255.
5. Holtmann B, Wray RC, Little AG. A randomized comparison of four incisions for orbital fractures. *Plast Reconstr Surg*. 1981;67:731.
6. Bahr W, Bagambisa FB, Schlegel G, et al. Comparison of transcutaneous incisions used for exposure of the infraorbital rim and orbital floor: a retrospective study. *Plast Reconstr Surg*. 1992;90:585.
7. Manson PN, Ruas E, Iliff N, et al. Single eyelid incision for exposure of the zygomatic bone and orbital reconstruction. *Plast Reconstr Surg*. 1987;79:120.

3 Transconjunctival Approaches

Transconjunctival approaches expose the floor of the orbit and infraorbital rim. More recently, these approaches have been extended medially to expose the medial wall of the orbit.

The significant advantage of transconjunctival approaches is that the scar is hidden in the conjunctiva. If a canthotomy is performed in conjunction with the approach, the only visible scar is the lateral extension, which heals leaving an inconspicuous scar. Transconjunctival techniques are rapid because neither skin nor muscle dissection is necessary. These simple techniques, however, demand surgical precision in execution because the complication of improper transconjunctival technique (i.e., entropion) is much more difficult to correct than the sequela of an improper skin incision (i.e., ectropion).

Another advantage of the transconjunctival approach is that the medial extent of the incision can be expanded superiorly, behind the lacrimal drainage system, as high as the levator aponeurosis. This approach has been called the *transcaruncular* because of the incision's relation to the caruncle. This approach can be useful when access to the medial orbital wall is required.

This chapter will discuss both approaches because they are often combined in practice.

Transconjunctival Approach to the Infraorbital Rim and Floor of the Orbit

The traditional transconjunctival incision, also called the *inferior fornix incision*, is a popular approach for exposing the orbital floor and infraorbital rim. Both preseptal and retroseptal approaches have been described. These approaches vary in the relation of the orbital septum to the path of dissection (see Fig. 3.1). The retroseptal approach is more direct than the preseptal approach and is easier to perform. An additional advantage is that there is no dissection within the eyelid, which may help avoid scarring within it. The periorbital fat may be encountered during the retroseptal approach, but this is of little concern and causes no ill effects. A lateral canthotomy enhances exposure and is frequently employed. The retroseptal transconjunctival approach with a lateral canthotomy is described in this chapter (Video 3.1).

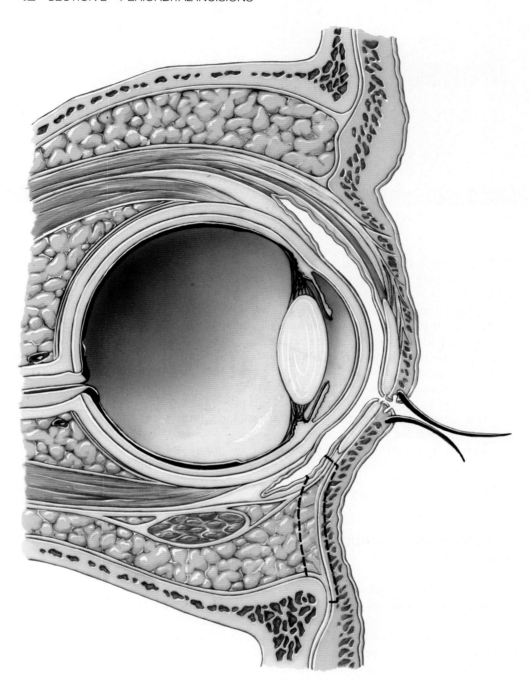

FIGURE 3.1 Sagittal section through orbit showing preseptal and retroseptal placement of incision.

Surgical Anatomy

Lower Eyelid

In addition to the anatomy described in Chapter 2, for the lower eyelid approach, the transconjunctival approach to the infraorbital rim and orbital floor requires the comprehension of other points.

Lower Eyelid Retractors During full downward gaze, the lower eyelid descends approximately 2 mm in conjunction with the movement of the globe itself. The inferior rectus muscle, which rotates the globe downward, simultaneously uses its fascial extension to retract the lower eyelid. This extension, which arises from the inferior rectus, contains sympathetic-innervated

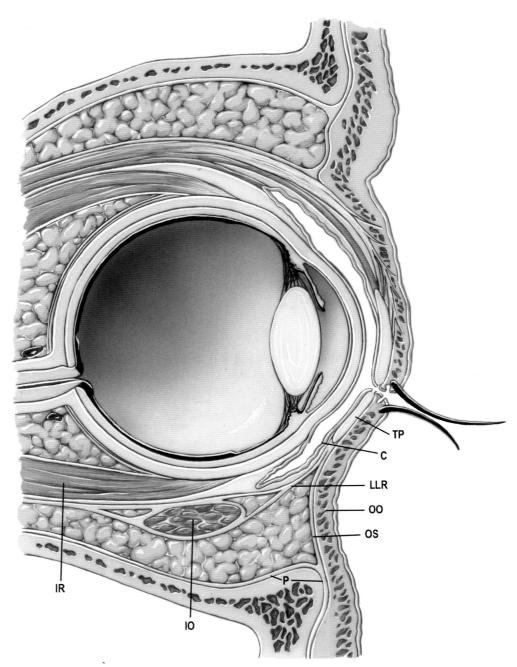

FIGURE 3.2 Sagittal section through orbit and globe. *C*, palpebral conjunctiva; *IO*, inferior oblique muscle; *IR*, inferior rectus muscle; *LLR*, lower lid retractors; *OO*, orbicularis oculi muscle; *OS*, orbital septum; *P*, periosteum/periorbita; *TP*, tarsal plate.

muscle fibers and is commonly called the *capsulopalpebral fascia* (see Fig. 3.2). Incision of this fascial sheet is clinically inconsequential when closure of the incision is correctly achieved.

Technique

➤ **STEP 1.** Vasoconstriction

A vasoconstrictor is injected under the conjunctiva to aid in hemostasis (see Fig. 3.3A). Additional solution is infiltrated during the lateral canthotomy (Fig. 3.3B).

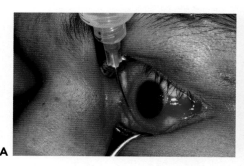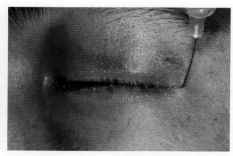

FIGURE 3.3 Photographs showing delivery of small amounts of local anesthetic with a vasoconstrictor, under the conjunctiva **(A)** and in the area of the lateral canthotomy **(B)**.

➤ **STEP 2.** Protection of the Globe

Because tarsorrhaphy is precluded with this approach, a corneal shield should be placed to protect the globe (see Fig. 3.4).

➤ **STEP 3.** Traction Sutures in the Lower Eyelid

The lower eyelid is everted with fine forceps and two or three traction sutures are placed through the eyelid (Fig. 3.4). These sutures should be placed straight through the eyelid, from palpebral conjunctiva to skin, approximately 4 to 5 mm below the eyelid margin to ensure that the tarsal plate is included in the suture.

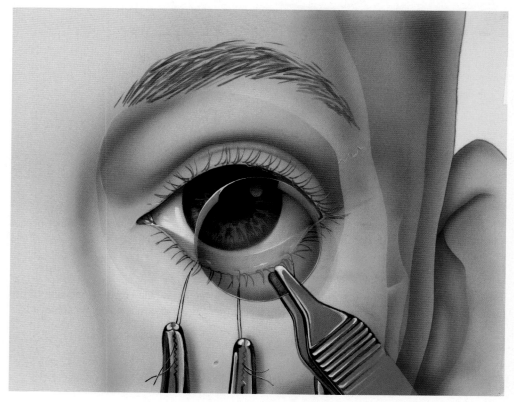

FIGURE 3.4 Placement of a corneal protector (shield). Two or three traction sutures placed through the lower eyelid assist in the placement of the shield and in subsequent surgery.

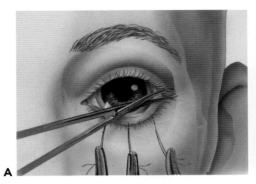
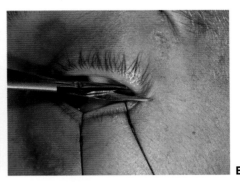

FIGURE 3.5 Illustration **(A)** and photograph **(B)** of initial incision for lateral canthotomy.

➤ **STEP 4.** Lateral Canthotomy and Inferior Cantholysis

When a lateral canthotomy is indicated, the canthotomy is the initial incision. One tip of the pointed scissors is inserted within the palpebral fissure, extending laterally to the depth of the underlying lateral orbital rim (approximately 7 to 10 mm). The scissors are used to cut horizontally through the lateral palpebral fissure (see Fig. 3.5). The structures that are cut in the horizontal plane are the skin, orbicularis oculi muscle, orbital septum, lateral canthal tendon, and conjunctiva.

The traction sutures are used to evert the lower eyelid. The lower eyelid is still tethered to the lateral orbital rim by the inferior limb of the lateral canthal tendon (see Fig. 3.6A). This tethering functionally adapts the lower eyelid tightly to the globe (Fig. 3.6B). The tendon, which is easily visualized with eyelid retraction, is released with a sharp vertical cut. To perform the cantholysis, the scissors must be positioned with a vertical orientation (see Fig. 3.7). After cantholysis (see Fig. 3.8A), the lower eyelid is immediately freed from the lateral orbital rim (Fig. 3.8B), making the eversion more effective.

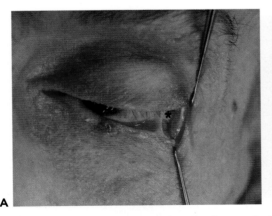
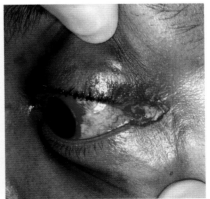

FIGURE 3.6 A: Anatomic dissection showing result after initial canthotomy illustrated in Figure 3.5. Note that the inferior limb of the lateral canthal tendon (*) is still attached to the lower tarsus, preventing mobilization. The lower eyelid is still tightly adapted to the eyeball **(B)**.

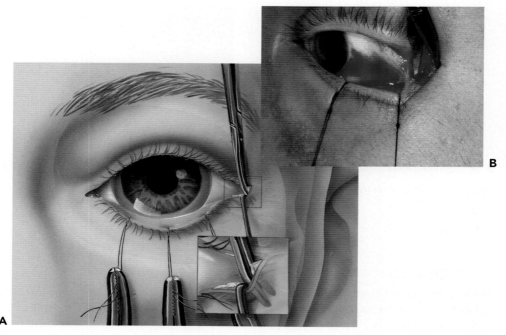

FIGURE 3.7 Illustration **(A)** and photograph **(B)** showing technique of inferior cantholysis.

➤ **STEP 5.** Transconjunctival Incision

After the lower eyelid is everted, the position of the lower tarsal plate through the conjunctiva is noted. One of two following techniques can be used to incise the conjunctiva. In the first technique, blunt-tipped pointed scissors are used to dissect through the small incision in the conjunctiva made during the lateral canthotomy, inferiorly toward the infraorbital rim. Traction sutures are used to evert the lower eyelid during the dissection. The scissors are spread to clear a pocket posterior to the orbital septum, ending just posterior to the orbital rim (see Fig. 3.9).

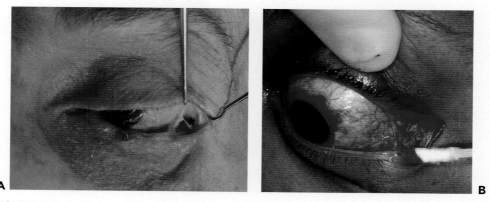

FIGURE 3.8 A: Anatomic dissection showing result after inferior cantholysis illustrated in Figure 3.7. Note that the inferior limb of the lateral canthal tendon (*) has been severed, allowing the lower eyelid great mobility **(B)**.

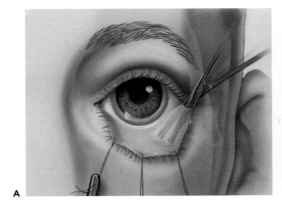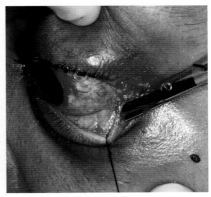

FIGURE 3.9 Illustration **(A)** and photograph **(B)** showing how the scissors are placed into the initial canthopexy incision to dissect in the subconjunctival plane. The dissection should be just below the tarsal plate and should extend no farther medially than the lacrimal punctum. Note how the traction sutures through the lower eyelid assist in this dissection.

Scissors are used to incise the conjunctiva and lower eyelid retractors midway between the inferior margin of the tarsal plate and the inferior conjunctival fornix (see Fig. 3.10). The incision can be extended as far medially as necessary for the surgery but must not violate the lacrimal sac.

The incised edge of the vestibular conjunctiva can be dissected free (see Fig. 3.11), providing a location for a traction suture to hold the corneal shield in place (see Fig. 3.12).

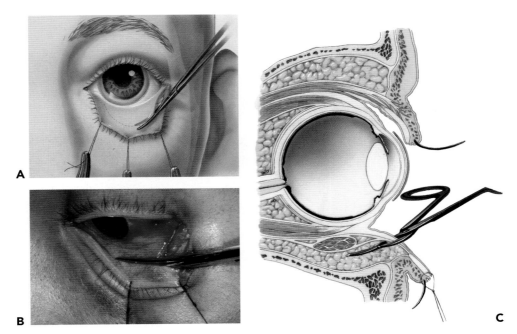

FIGURE 3.10 Illustration **(A)** and photograph **(B)** showing incision of the conjunctiva below the tarsal plate. **C:** Sagittal plane through the orbit and globe demonstrating the level and plane of incision. The conjunctiva and lower eyelid retractors are incised with scissors.

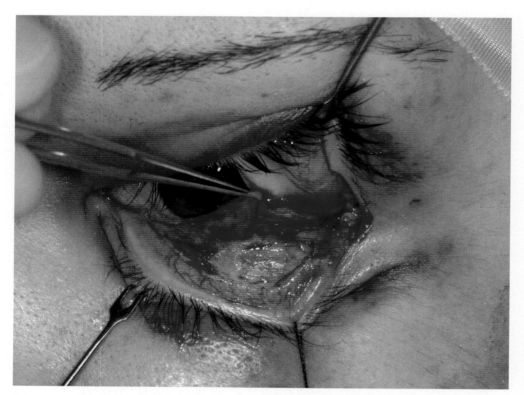

FIGURE 3.11 The incised edge of the vestibular conjunctiva is dissected free so that a traction suture can be placed.

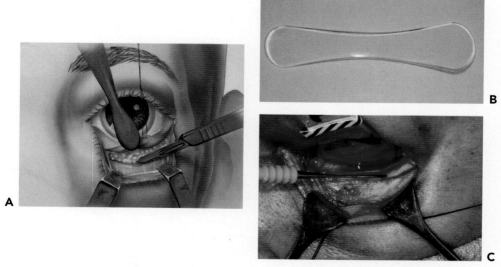

FIGURE 3.12 A: Illustration showing incision through the periorbita. Small retractors are placed so that the lower eyelid is retracted to the level of the anterior surface of the infraorbital rim. A broad retractor is placed just posterior to the infraorbital rim, confining the orbital fat. The Jaeger Lid Plate (Jaeger Lid Plates—Anthony Products, Inc., Indianapolis, IN) is a clear plastic retractor **(B)** that works well for retracting the orbital contents because it is transparent. The incision is made through the periosteum just posterior to the infraorbital rim with either a scalpel or electrocautery **(C)**.

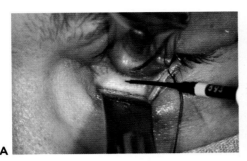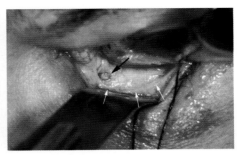

A   **B**

FIGURE 3.13 Photographs showing another method of incising the conjunctiva. With the lower eyelid retracted anteriorly, a fine-tipped electrocautery is used to incise the conjunctiva **(A)**. (In this instance, a lateral canthotomy was not performed.) Once the conjunctiva is incised **(B)** (*white arrows*), the electrocautery is used to incise the lower eyelid retractors and periorbita (*black arrow*).

➤ **STEP 6.** Periosteal Incision

After retracting the orbital contents internally and the lower eyelid externally, using suitable retractors, the periorbita is sharply incised, avoiding the lacrimal sac medially (Fig. 3.12). During the retroseptal approach, the incision through the periorbita is immediately posterior to the orbital rim.

An alternate method of incising the conjunctiva, lower eyelid retractors, and periorbita incorporates retracting the lower eyelid anteriorly, inserting small retractors, and cutting directly through these structures with a needle-tipped electrocautery (see Fig. 3.13).

➤ **STEP 7.** Subperiosteal Orbital Dissection

Periosteal elevators are used to strip the periosteum over the orbital rim and anterior surface of the maxilla and zygoma, and the orbital floor (see Fig. 3.14). A broad malleable retractor should be placed as soon as feasible to protect the orbit and to confine any herniating periorbital fat.

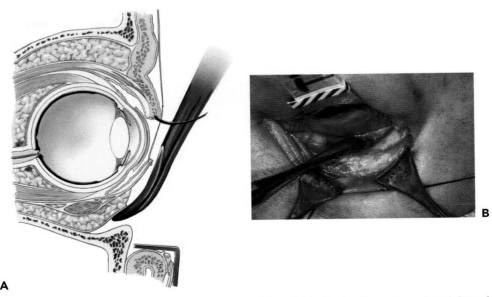

A   **B**

FIGURE 3.14 Subperiosteal dissection of the orbital floor. Note the traction suture placed through the cut end of the conjunctiva **(A)**, which assists in retracting the conjunctiva and maintains the corneal shield in place. **B:** Photograph showing use of periosteal elevator to strip the periosteum from the orbital floor. Note the clear retractor used to elevate the tissues.

➤ **STEP 8.** Closure

Periosteal suturing is not mandatory but optional, if exposure permits. Before closing the conjunctiva, an inferior canthopexy suture is inserted but not tied (see Fig. 3.15). Delaying the tying of this suture allows open access to the conjunctiva for its closure. If the conjunctiva were to be closed first, the sutures might tear through the delicate tissue during the inferior canthopexy.

A 4-0 polyglactin or other long-lasting suture is used to reattach the lateral portion of the inferior tarsal plate to the residual superior portion of the lateral canthal tendon or to the fixed surrounding tissues. This suture should be securely located in the appropriate anatomic location so that the lateral canthal area appears symmetrical to the contralateral eye and the eyelid is adjacent to the globe. When the inferior limb of the canthal tendon is initially severed during the approach, only a minute amount of canthal tendon remains attached to the lower tarsus. Therefore, the canthopexy anchor suture may be inserted through the lateral border of the tarsus only when the tendon is inadequate to retain a suture. The suture through the lateral border of the lower tarsus and/or cut portion of the lateral canthal tendon may be facilitated by elevating the skin sharply with a blade, slightly atop the canthus or tarsal plate. This is easily performed by using a no. 15 scalpel to incise between the tarsus and the skin. A cleavage plane exists in this location, and the tissue readily separates. The tarsus is grasped with forceps and a suture is passed through either the cut tendon or the lateral border of the tarsus in such a manner that a firm bite of tissue is engaged (Fig. 3.15A and B). After a good bite of the lower tarsus has been secured with the suture, the suture needle is inserted through the superior limb of the lateral canthal tendon and/or the periosteum of the lateral orbital rim in the vertex of the palpebral fissure.

The bulk of the lateral canthal tendon attaches to the orbital tubercle, 3 to 4 mm *posterior* to the orbital margin. Following canthotomy, the superior limb of the canthal tendon is still attached to the orbital tubercle. The suture should be inserted as deeply behind the orbital rim as possible to adapt the lower eyelid to the globe. If the suture is not properly

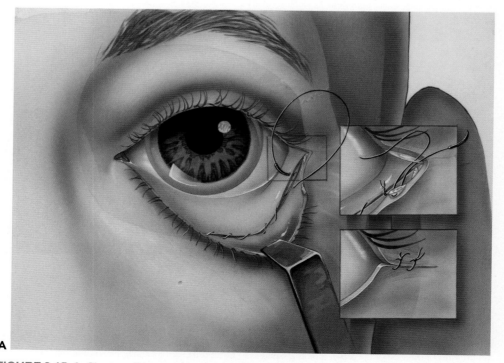

A

FIGURE 3.15 A: Closure of transconjunctival incision and inferior canthopexy. The inferior canthopexy suture is placed (***upper inset***).

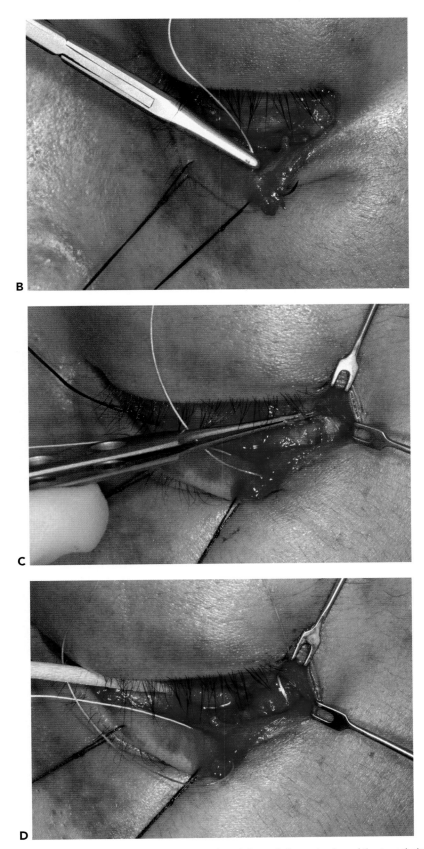

FIGURE 3.15 (*continued*) **B:** A suture has been placed through the cut edge of the tarsal plate of the lower eyelid. **C:** Forceps are used to identify the superior portion of the lateral canthal tendon. **D:** The suture is placed through the superior canthal tendon.   (*continued*)

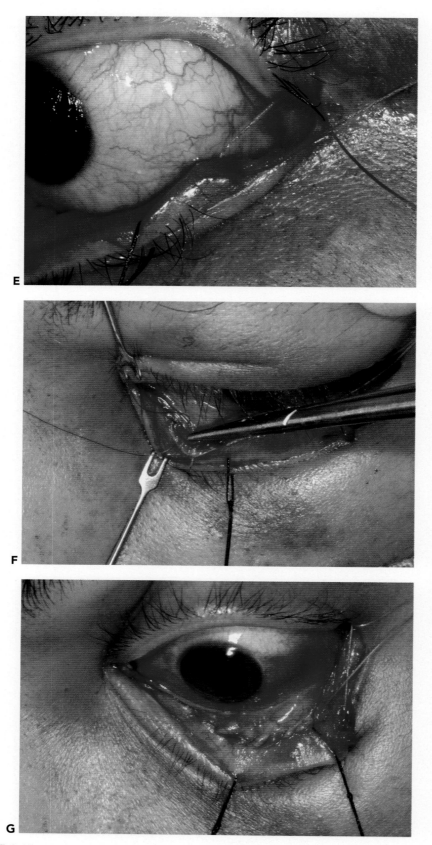

FIGURE 3.15 (*continued*) **E:** The suture is not tied but left lax. **F:** Closure of the conjunctiva and lower eyelid retractors **G:** Appearance after closure of the conjunctiva and just prior to tying the inferior canthopexy suture.

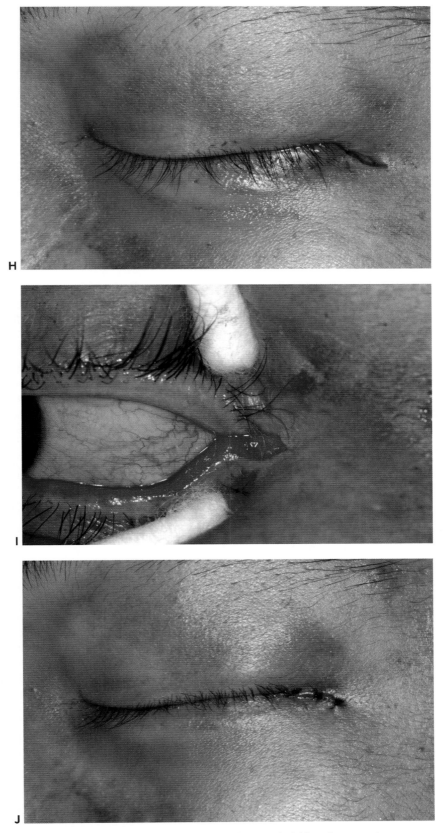

FIGURE 3.15 (*continued*) **H:** Appearance after canthopexy tied. Note the normal appearance to the lateral aspect of the palpebral fissure. **I:** Separation of the tissues with cotton-tipped applicators shows the lower eyelid reapproximated. **J:** Skin sutured.

placed, the eyelid will not contact the globe laterally, and will give an unnatural appearance. Therefore, the suture needle should be passed far posteriorly and superiorly to ensure that it grasps the superior limb of the tendon. An effective method is to first identify the superior limb of the canthal tendon by placing a small, toothed forceps within the incision (Fig. 3.15C). The forceps is then passed along the medial side of the lateral orbital rim for a few millimeters until the dense fibers of the superior limb are located. While the tendon is being held, the suture needle should be passed through the tendon (Fig. 3.15D). The two ends of the suture should be pulled to ensure that the suture is firmly attached, or pexed, to ligamentous tissue. The suture should be left untied until the conjunctiva has been closed (Fig. 3.15E).

The conjunctiva should be closed with a running 6-0 chromic gut suture (Fig. 3.15F and G). The ends of the suture may be buried. No attempt should be made to reapproximate the lower eyelid retractors because they are in intimate contact with the conjunctiva and will be adequately repositioned when that layer is closed.

The inferior canthopexy suture is then tightened and tied, drawing the lower eyelid into position (Fig. 3.15H and I).

Finally, subcutaneous sutures and 6-0 skin sutures are placed along the horizontal lateral canthotomy (Fig. 3.15J).

Alternative Technique: Extended Transconjunctival Approach for Exposure of the Frontozygomatic Area

The extended transconjunctival approach provides access to the entire lateral orbital rim to a point approximately 10 to 12 mm superior to the frontozygomatic suture. For this added exposure, however, a more generous lateral canthotomy incision and wider undermining are needed. Additionally, the superior limb of the lateral canthal tendon must be stripped from its insertions. The approach is useful when access to the entire lateral orbit, lateral orbital rim, orbital floor, and inferior orbital rim is required.

The incision for the extended transconjunctival approach is exactly as described for the standard transconjunctival approach, but the incision must be extended further laterally, 1 to 1.5 cm in a natural crease. If no natural skin crease extends laterally from the lateral palpebral fissure, the extension can usually be made straight laterally or slightly superolaterally.

Supraperiosteal dissection of the entire lateral orbital rim is performed to a point above the frontozygomatic suture. The orbicularis oculi musculature and superficial portion of the lateral canthal tendon are retracted as the dissection proceeds.

After retraction, the periosteum is incised in the middle of the lateral orbital rim from the highest point obtained with supraperiosteal dissection. The periosteal incision extends to the one described from the standard approach to the orbital floor and infraorbital rim. Subperiosteal dissection should strip all the tissues from the orbital floor and the lateral orbital wall. Generous subperiosteal dissection made deep into the lateral orbit allows retraction of these tissues to expose the frontozygomatic suture (see Fig. 3.16).

This extent of exposure and release demands meticulous closure, with anatomical resuspension of tissues and the lateral canthus within the orbit.

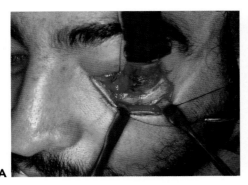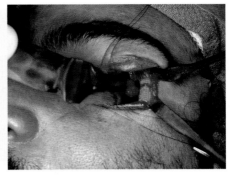

FIGURE 3.16 Photographs showing the amount of exposure that can be attained from the extended transconjunctival approach. **A:** Exposure of the orbital floor. **B:** Exposure of the lateral wall of the orbit, as well as the frontozygomatic suture.

Transconjunctival (or Transcaruncular) Approach to the Medial Orbit

The medial wall of the orbit can be approached through the conjunctiva on the nasal side of the globe. This approach has been most commonly called the "transcaruncular" approach because the caruncle is traversed with the initial incision. Others, however, place the incision just temporal to the caruncle.

There are no vulnerable structures in the medial orbit with the transcaruncular approach from the 11:00 position of the globe of the left eye where the trochlea and levator aponeurosis are encountered to the 6:00 position where the inferior oblique muscle is encountered. Therefore, even though the initial access incision may only be 12 mm, access may be extended subperiosteally to the orbital roof and the infraorbital rim (Video 3.2).

The advantage of the transconjunctival approach to the medial orbit is avoiding a local skin incision or a coronal approach to reach this area. The access provided is satisfactory for most reconstructive procedures. By extending the transconjunctival incision along the floor of the orbit, complete exposure of the medial wall, floor, and lateral wall of the orbit is possible through a single incision.

Surgical Anatomy

The anatomy of the medial aspect of the orbit underlying the transcaruncular approach is complex but most of it can be avoided when the dissection is executed properly. The medial canthal tendon is the centerpiece of medial canthal anatomy. It has an elastic lateral portion that supports the lacrimal canaliculi and then splits into anterior, superior, and posterior limbs, all of which blend with the lacrimal sac fascia (see Chapter 2).

The preseptal portion of the orbicularis oculi muscle has a superficial head and a deep head. The superficial head originates from the anterior limb of the medial canthal tendon. The deep head originates from the fascia of the lacrimal sac. The pretarsal portion of the orbicularis oculi muscle sends anterior fibers to the anterior portion of the medial canthal tendon and posterior fibers that line the posterior wall of the lacrimal sac to insert on the posterior lacrimal crest (lacrimal bone) (see Fig. 3.17). These posterior fibers form an especially important structure known as the *pars lacrimalis* or *Horner muscle* and ensure proper posterior apposition of the eyelid to the globe. Disruption of Horner muscle might allow the medial eyelid to fall anteriorly away from the globe.

Between the anterior and posterior limbs of the medial canthal tendons lies the lacrimal sac into which tears drain from the canaliculi. This region is known as the *lacrimal sac fossa* and is bordered by the bony anterior and posterior lacrimal crests (Fig. 3.17). Inferiorly, the fossa is contiguous with the bony nasolacrimal duct. Superiorly, the lacrimal sac extends just slightly above the medial canthal tendon.

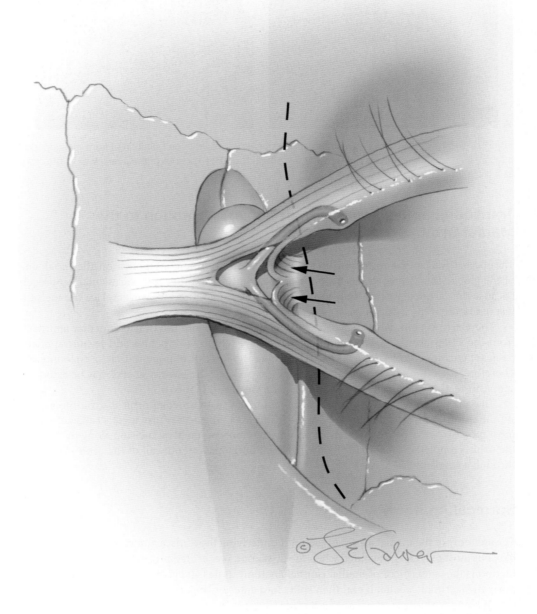

FIGURE 3.17 Illustration showing the relation of the periosteal incision of the orbit (*dashed line*), the osteology, the edges of the eyelids, the lacrimal drainage system, and Horner muscle (*arrows*). The incision through the periosteum is posterior to all the structures shown.

Surface anatomy is especially important in the transcaruncular approach to the medial orbit (see Fig. 3.18). The plica semilunaris (semilunar fold) is a narrow, highly vascularized, crescent-shaped fold of the medial conjunctiva. Its lateral border is free and is separated from the bulbar conjunctiva. The caruncle is a small, fleshy, keratinized mound of sebaceous tissue attached to the inferomedial side of the plica semilunaris. Just medial to it lies the common canaliculus.

A condensation of fascia exists deep to the caruncle. It is continuous with the medial canthal ligament, and serves as the anterior insertion for several structures, including Horner muscle, the medial orbital septum, the medial capsulopalpebral muscle, and the anterior

Tenon capsule. Horner muscle and the medial orbital septum insert into the periorbita immediately posterior to the posterior lacrimal crest. The anatomic plane in which these fascial extensions lie is a potential region for surgical dissection that avoids the medial rectus muscle posteriorly and laterally and the lacrimal drainage system anteriorly and medially. An incision made through the caruncle and this dense fibrous condensation passes along a natural plane just posterior to Horner muscle, which buffers this safe and bloodless plane from the lacrimal sac.

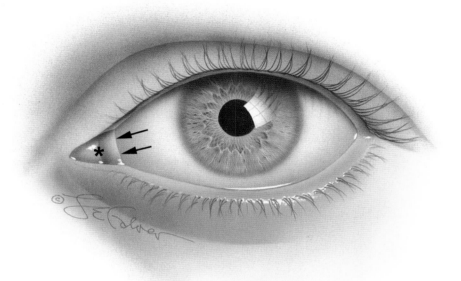

A

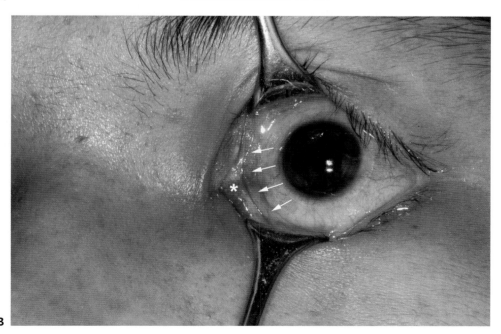

B

FIGURE 3.18 Illustration **(A)** and photograph **(B)** showing the surface topography of the eye. The "*" is the location of the caruncle. The *arrows* indicate the position of the semilunar fold.   (*continued*)

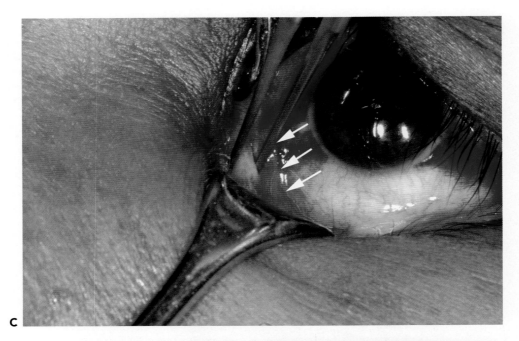

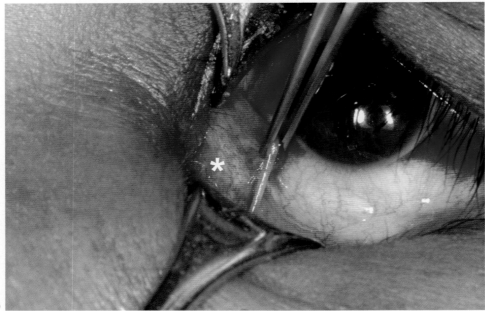

FIGURE 3.18 (*continued*) **C:** Forceps are grasping the caruncle. **D:** Forceps are lifting the semilunar fold. The "*" is the location of the caruncle.

Technique

➤ **STEP 1.** Vasoconstriction

The medial orbit is infiltrated with a vasoconstrictor to facilitate hemostasis. The solution is delivered to the medial orbit through the conjunctiva or through the skin just nasal to the eyelids. The conjunctiva in the area of the caruncle and semilunar fold can be infiltrated, but doing so can distort these structures and make incision location difficult. If one decides to infiltrate the conjunctiva, 7 to 10 minutes should pass to allow the solution to diffuse peripherally.

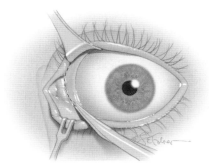
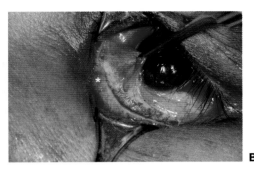

A   **B**

FIGURE 3.19 Incision through the medial conjunctiva. **A:** Illustration showing the use of scissors to make the incision. Note the position of the caruncle and semilunar folds in relation to the incision, which is just lateral to the caruncle. **B:** Photograph showing incision that has been made with needle-point cautery. The forces are grasping and retracting the semilunar fold. The "*" is the position of the caruncle.

➤ **STEP 2.** Transconjunctival Incision

The upper and lower eyelids are retracted with traction sutures, vein retractors, or Desmarres retractors, taking care to avoid damage to the lacrimal puncta and canaliculi. The globe is retracted laterally by inserting a malleable Jaeger Lid Plate retractor into the medial fornix. This increases the distance between the posterior surface of the eyelids and the globe, facilitating ease of incision. Gentle pressure is given posteriorly on the globe with this retractor to protect the globe from inadvertent incision, flatten the caruncle, increase the visibility of the area of incision, and force the extraconal orbital fat posteriorly in this area.

It is important to avoid the semilunar fold, which is lateral to the caruncle. A 12-to 15-mm vertical incision is made through the conjunctiva and lateral one third of the caruncle using Stevens or Westcott scissors (see Fig. 3.19). Alternatively, the incision can be made just temporal to the caruncle. The incision can be made superiorly through the conjunctiva to the level of the levator palpebrae aponeurosis.

➤ **STEP 3.** Subconjunctival Dissection

The condensed fibrous layer just deep to the caruncle is dissected in a posteromedial direction, aiming just posterior to the posterior lacrimal crest. Horner muscle provides a natural plane for dissection down to the posterior lacrimal crest, where it inserts. The tips of the curved Stevens scissors (see Fig. 3.20) or a Freer elevator are used to palpate the posterior lacrimal crest. The tips of the instrument can be rolled anteroposteriorly to help identify the posterior

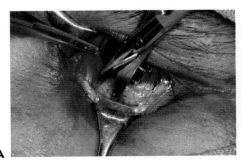
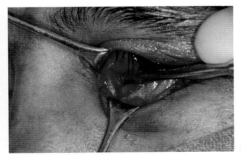

A   **B**

FIGURE 3.20 Dissection deep to the conjunctiva. **A:** Photograph showing the use of scissors to spread into the conjunctival incision toward the medial orbital wall. The points of the scissors or a Freer elevator **(B)** can be used to palpate the posterior lacrimal crest to ensure that the dissection is posterior to it and to the Horner muscle.

lacrimal crest. The dissection should be performed on the posterior side of the posterior lacrimal crest. A malleable retractor or periosteal elevator is held firmly against the medial orbital wall immediately posterior to the posterior lacrimal crest. This establishes the plane of the dissection, which is then performed with scissors. The scissors are spread gently to expose the periorbita immediately posterior to the posterior lacrimal crest. The plane of dissection passes along the posterior aspect of Horner muscle. After the scissors have been spread to expose the medial orbit, a malleable retractor is inserted before removing the scissors.

➤ **STEP 4.** Periosteal Incision and Exposure

The periorbita along the posterior lacrimal crest is incised in a superior to inferior direction with a scalpel or a needle cautery, or with a spreading motion of sharp, pointed scissors (see Fig. 3.21). This incision should be just posterior to the insertion of Horner muscle onto the posterior lacrimal crest. Subperiosteal dissection of the medial wall begins with a periosteal elevator. The periorbita is elevated superiorly and inferiorly to obtain a wide anterior aperture. The medial wall of the orbit is exposed from the floor to the roof (see Fig. 3.22). The anterior and posterior ethmoidal arteries are readily identified, cauterized, and cut. A malleable retractor is placed deep along the medial wall and, when retracted, the medial wall is exposed.

➤ **STEP 5.** Closure

Closure of the periorbita is not essential and is quite difficult to perform. It is prudent to repair the conjunctiva and the caruncle with 6-0 gut suture to help prevent symblepharon, pyogenic granuloma, and orbital fat prolapse.

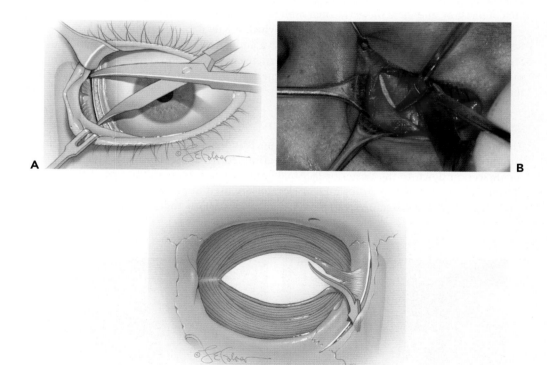

FIGURE 3.21 Periosteal incision. Illustration **(A)** and photograph **(B)** showing the use of scissors to open the periosteum along the medial orbital wall. **C:** Illustration from within the left orbit facing externally, showing the path of dissection. Note the periosteal incision is made posterior to the Horner muscle.

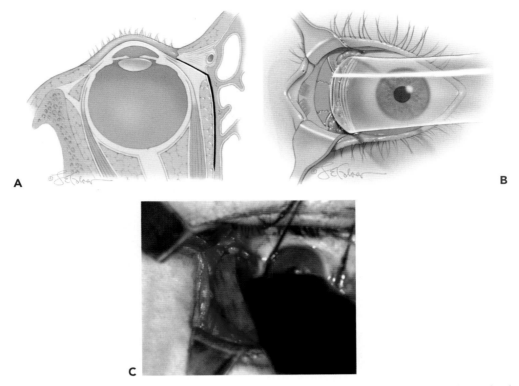

FIGURE 3.22 Exposure of the medial wall of the orbit. **A:** Illustration demonstrating the path of dissection along the medial orbital wall. Illustration **(B)** and photograph **(C)** showing the medial wall exposed.

Combining Transconjunctival Approaches

The transcaruncular approach can be used for isolated medial orbital wall surgery or combined with a retroseptal transconjunctival approach to the orbital floor (with or without a lateral canthotomy; see preceding text). By so doing, the entire medial wall, medial floor, and lateral wall of the orbit can be exposed.

When combined with a transconjunctival approach to the floor of the orbit, lateral canthotomy and inferior cantholysis are done first (see preceding text). The lower eyelid is retracted anteriorly and inferiorly to provide improved access to the medial conjunctival surfaces (see Fig. 3.23A). Scissors are then used to first undermine (Fig. 3.23B) and then to incise the conjunctiva just lateral to the caruncle (Fig. 3.23C). The incision is continued superiorly to the level of the levator aponeurosis (Fig. 3.23D).

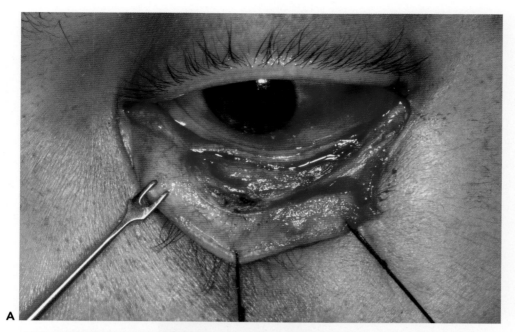

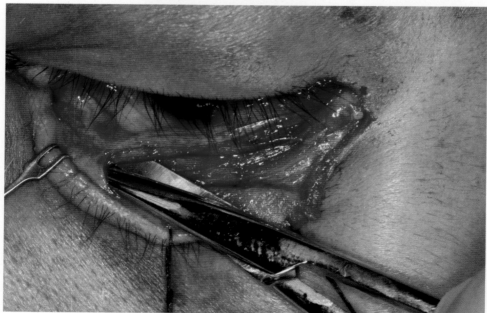

FIGURE 3.23 Photographs showing the medial transconjunctival approach combined with a standard transconjunctival approach to the orbital floor. **A:** Lateral canthotomy, inferior cantholysis, and incision through the conjunctiva have been performed. Note that the lower eyelid can be retracted anteriorly to provide access to the medial aspect of the fornix. **B:** Undermining of conjunctiva medial to the globe.

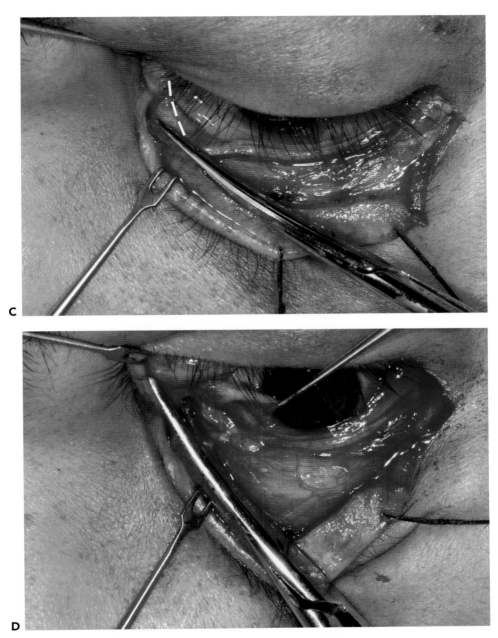

FIGURE 3.23 (*continued*) **C:** Incising the conjunctiva just lateral to the caruncle with scissors. **D:** Extending the conjunctival incision superiorly along the medial aspect of the orbit.

During the dissection, the inferior oblique muscle is encountered (see Fig. 3.24A). This muscle can either be stripped from its origin or severed from its bony attachment (Fig. 3.24B). If it is incised, leaving a small amount of muscle still attached to the bone, a single suture can be placed during closure to reapproximate the severed muscle. If it is stripped from its origin, it does not have to be repositioned. One can then continue the incision and dissection supero-medially as described earlier in this chapter.

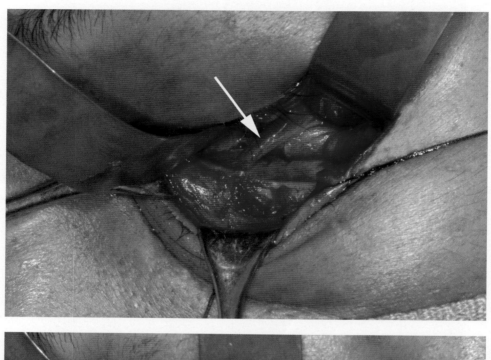

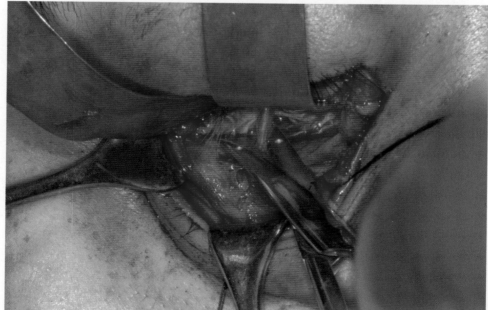

FIGURE 3.24 Photographs showing the inferior oblique muscle (**A**, *arrow*). Scissors are shown incising this muscle (**B**).

4 Supraorbital Eyebrow Approach

Surgical Anatomy

The "in the eyebrow" incision offers simple and rapid camouflaged access to the lateral supraorbital rim, the frontozygomatic suture line, and occasionally the region slightly below it. No important neurovascular structures are involved in this approach. If the incision is to be continued along the lateral orbit for more inferior exposure, the incision crosses the resting skin tension lines or crow's feet perpendicularly; therefore, this option should be avoided. Additionally, cosmetic eyebrow removal restricts this incision for women. For these reasons, the supraorbital eyebrow approach is not recommended, except possibly for men whose fracture lines are high on the lateral orbital rim. The main disadvantages of the approach are the extremely limited access it provides and a scar that is perceptible within the eyebrow or, if extended inferiorly, below it.

A previously popular incision used to gain access to the superolateral orbital rim is the eyebrow incision. Apart from the advantage that this approach involves no important neurovascular structures, it gives simple and rapid access to the frontozygomatic area. If the incision is made almost entirely within the confines of the eyebrow, the scar is usually imperceptible. Occasionally, however, there is some hair loss, which makes the scar perceptible. Unfortunately, this approach is undesirable in individuals whose eyebrows are not extended laterally and inferiorly along the orbital margin. Incisions made along the lateral orbital rim outside the eyebrow are very conspicuous in such individuals, for whom another type of incision may be indicated. The main disadvantage of the approach is its extremely limited access (Video 4.1).

Technique

➤ STEP 1. Vasoconstriction

A local anesthetic along with a vasoconstrictor is injected into the subcutaneous tissues over the lateral orbital rim to aid in hemostasis.

➤ STEP 2. Skin Incision

The eyebrow is not shaved. The skin is straddled over the orbital rim using two fingers, and an incision of 2 cm or longer is made, with the inferior extent of the incision arresting at the end of the eyebrow. The incision is made parallel to the hair of the eyebrow to avoid cutting the hair shafts. The incision is extended up to the depth of the periosteum (see Fig. 4.1). The skin is freely movable in this plane.

Access can be improved by extending the incision more anteriorly within the confines of the eyebrow to the supraorbital nerve. Extending the incision inferiorly along the orbital rim should be avoided because the incision would cross the lines of resting skin tension, making

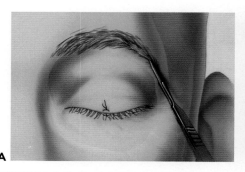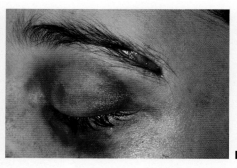

FIGURE 4.1 Illustration showing placement of incision within confines of eyebrow hair **(A)**. The incision is made through the skin and subcutaneous tissues to the level of the periosteum in one stroke. Note that the entire incision is within the confines of the hair of the eyebrow **(B)**.

the scar very conspicuous. When indicated, extension of the incision inferiorly may utilize a small gentle 90-degree "skin-only" turn into a crow's foot wrinkle laterally. High extensions must avoid the frontal branch of the facial nerve and low extensions should be at least 6 mm above the level of the lateral canthus.

➤ **STEP 3.** Periosteal Incision

After undermining in the supraperiosteal plane, the skin is retracted over the area of interest where a sharp periosteal incision is made (see Fig. 4.2).

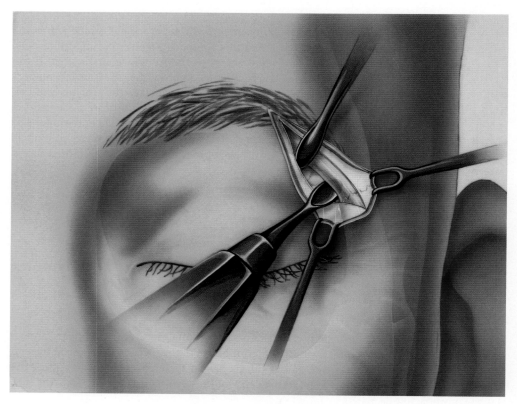

FIGURE 4.2 Incision through periosteum along lateral orbital rim and subperiosteal dissection into lacrimal fossa. Because of the concavity just behind the orbital rim in this area, the periosteal elevator is oriented laterally as dissection proceeds posteriorly.

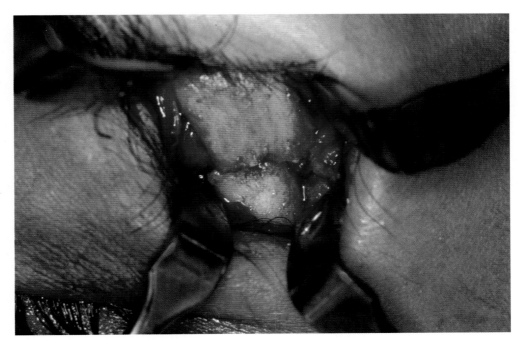

FIGURE 4.3 Photograph showing the limited extent of exposure provided by this approach when the incision is kept within the confines of the eyebrow.

➤ **STEP 4.** Subperiosteal Dissection of Lateral Orbital Rim and Lateral Orbit

Two sharp periosteal elevators are used to expose the lateral orbital rim on the lateral, medial (intraorbital), and if necessary, posterior (temporal) surfaces (Fig. 4.2). Wide undermining of the skin and periosteum allows the tissues to be retracted inferiorly, providing better access to the lower portions of the lateral orbital rim. However, the access provided by this approach is limited (see Fig. 4.3). If one stays within the subperiosteal space, there is virtually no possibility of damaging vital structures.

➤ **STEP 5.** Closure

The incision is closed in layers.

5 | Upper Eyelid Approach

The most direct and cosmetically appealing approach to the superolateral orbital rim is the upper eyelid approach, also called *upper blepharoplasty*, upper eyelid crease, and supratarsal fold approach. In this approach, a natural skin crease in the upper eyelid is used to make the incision (Video 5.1).

Surgical Anatomy

Upper Eyelid

In sagittal section, the upper eyelid consists of at least five distinct layers: the skin, the orbicularis oculi muscle, the orbital septum above or levator palpebrae superioris aponeurosis below, Müller muscle/tarsus complex, and the conjunctiva (see Fig. 5.1). The skin, orbicularis oculi muscle, and conjunctiva of the upper eyelid are similar to those of the lower eyelid (see Chapter 2). The upper eyelid differs from the lower eyelid, however, by the presence of the levator palpebral superioris aponeurosis and Müller muscle.

Orbital Septum/Levator Aponeurosis Complex Deep to the orbicularis oculi muscle lies the orbital septum/levator aponeurosis complex. Unlike the situation in the lower eyelid, where the orbital septum inserts into the tarsal plate, in the upper eyelid it extends inferiorly and blends with the levator aponeurosis approximately 10 to 15 mm above the upper eyelid margin. The levator muscle usually becomes aponeurotic at the equator of the globe in the superior orbit. The aponeurosis courses anteriorly to insert onto the anterior surface of the lower two thirds of the tarsal plate. Extensions of the levator aponeurosis also extend anteriorly into the skin of the lower portion of the upper eyelid. The aponeurotic portion of the levator behind the orbital septum is much wider than the muscle from which it is derived, and its medial and lateral extensions are known as *horns* or *cornua*. The lateral horn of the levator is prominent and deeply indents the anterior portion of the lacrimal gland to divide it into thin palpebral and thick orbital portions; its lateral extension attaches to the orbital wall at the orbital (Whitnall) tubercle. The weaker medial horn of the levator aponeurosis blends with the orbital septum and the medial check ligament.

Müller Muscle/Tarsus Complex Deep to the levator aponeurosis the Müller muscle lies superiorly while the tarsus lies along the eyelid margin. Müller muscle is a nonstriated, sympathetically innervated elevator of the upper eyelid. It originates from the inner surface of the levator aponeurosis and inserts onto the superior surface of the upper tarsal plate. The *tarsal plate* of the upper eyelid is a thin, pliable fibrocartilaginous structure that

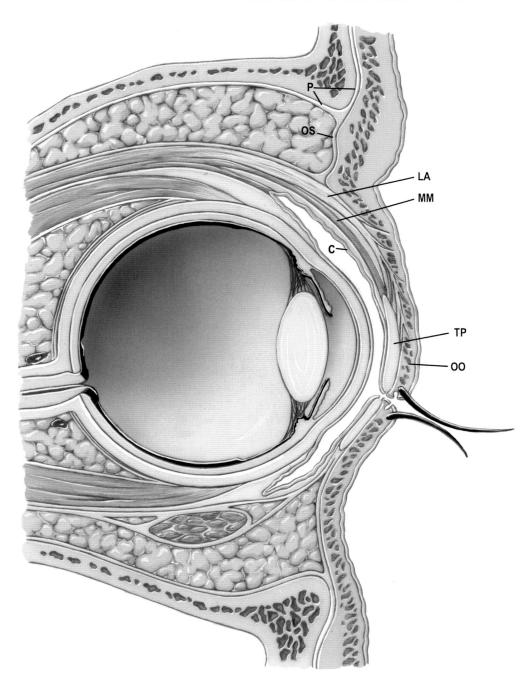

FIGURE 5.1 Sagittal section through orbit and globe. *C*, palpebral conjunctiva; *LA*, levator palpebral superioris aponeurosis; *MM*, Müller muscle; *OO*, orbicularis oculi muscle; *OS*, orbital septum; *P*, periosteum/periorbita; *TP*, tarsal plate.

gives form and support to the upper eyelid. Embedded within the tarsal plate are large sebaceous glands—the *tarsal* or *Meibomian glands.* The edge of the tarsus adjacent to the free border of the eyelid is parallel to it, whereas the deeper (superior) border is curved such that the tarsus is somewhat semilunar in shape. It is also curved to conform to the outer surface of the eyeball. The superior tarsus is considerably larger than the inferior tarsus, the greatest height of the superior tarsus being approximately 10 mm and that of the inferior tarsus being approximately 4 to 5 mm (see Fig. 2.6A and B). The tarsal glands sandwiched between the layers of fibrocartilage in the upper eyelid exit on the eyelid margin near the eyelash follicles. The eyelashes are supported by their roots, attached to fibrous tissue on the tarsal plate, not in the orbicularis oculi muscle anterior to the tarsal plate. Laterally, the tarsal plate becomes a fibrous band that adjoins the structural counterpart from the lower eyelid, forming the lateral canthal tendon. Medially, the tarsal plate also becomes fibrous and shelters the superior lacrimal canaliculus behind as it becomes the medial canthal tendon.

Technique

➤ STEP 1. Protection of the Globe

During surgical procedures around the orbit, the cornea should be protected with a temporary tarsorrhaphy or scleral shell after application of a bland eye ointment.

➤ STEP 2. Identification and Marking of Incision Line

If an eyelid crease is not readily detectable, a curvilinear incision along the area of the supratarsal fold that tails off laterally over the lateral orbital rim is made. Remarkably, the incision in the upper eyelid follows *either* the lower *or* the upper component of a standard blepharoplasty. In case of swelling, the opposite upper eyelid crease may be mirrored. The incision should be similar in location and shape to the lateral one third to one half of the superior incision in a blepharoplasty (see Fig. 5.2). The incision, however, may be extended farther laterally as necessary for surgical access. The incision should begin at least 10 mm superior to the upper eyelid margin and should be 6 mm above the lateral canthus as it extends laterally. The incision line is marked *before* infiltration of a vasoconstrictor to avoid distortion.

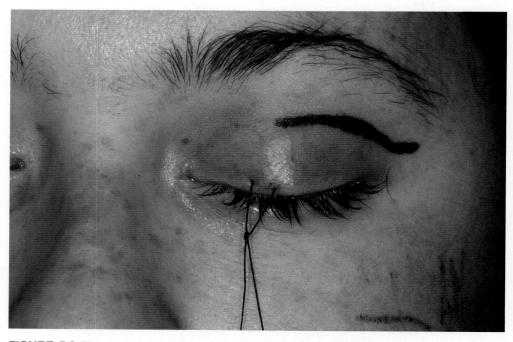

FIGURE 5.2 Photograph showing position of skin incision. The incision may be extended farther laterally if necessary.

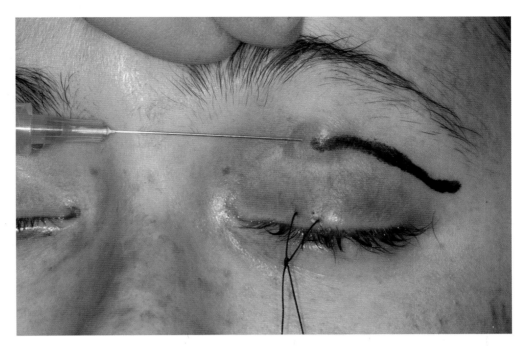

FIGURE 5.3 Photograph showing injection of local anesthetic with a vasoconstrictor under the orbicularis oculi muscle.

➤ **STEP 3.** Vasoconstriction

Local anesthesia with a vasoconstrictor is injected under the eyelid skin and the orbicularis oculi muscle along the incision line (see Fig. 5.3). Additional vasoconstrictor solution is injected supraperiosteally in the area to be surgically exposed.

➤ **STEP 4.** Skin Incision

Ideally, the incision cuts through both skin and orbicularis oculi muscle (see Fig. 5.4). In practice, it is often easier to perform the incision in the skin followed by dissection through the orbicularis oculi muscle with scissors (see Fig. 5.5). The vasculature of the muscle maintains the viability of the skin when they are elevated together, and this leads to excellent healing.

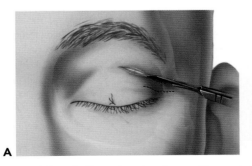
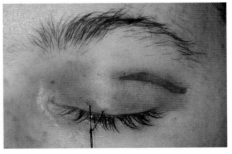

FIGURE 5.4 A: Illustration showing position and placement of the initial incision through the skin and orbicularis muscle. This illustration shows the position of the incision, which is similar to that of the upper incision during blepharoplasty. The (*dashed line*) below the first is an alternate position that can be used. This position is similar to a lower blepharoplasty incision. **B:** Photograph showing the initial incision made through the skin and some of the thickness of the orbicularis oculi muscle, which can be of variable thickness in this region.

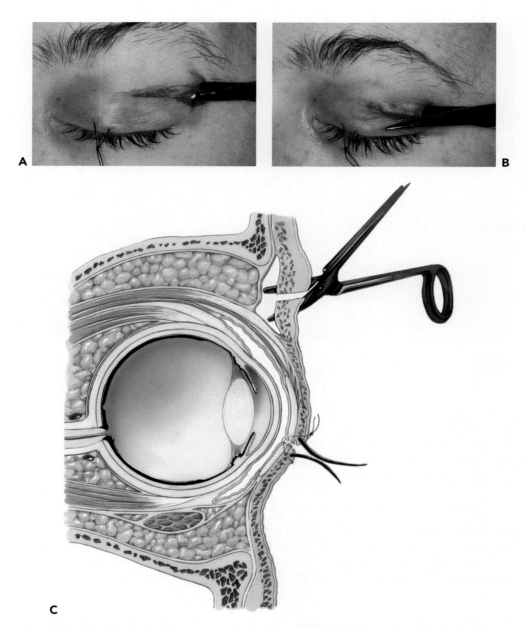

FIGURE 5.5 Photographs showing dissection through remaining orbicularis oculi muscle. The scissors are first used to spread underneath the muscle **(A)** and then to incise it **(B)**. Sagittal section through orbit and globe **(C)** showing dissection between orbicularis oculi muscle and the levator aponeurosis below and orbital septum above.

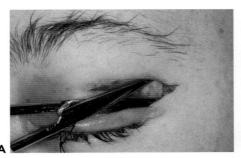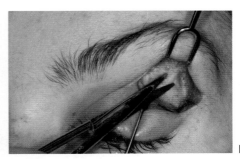

FIGURE 5.6 Photographs showing the use of scissors to dissect deep to the orbicularis oculi muscle plane toward the supraorbital and lateral orbital rims **(A)**. **B:** The supraperiosteal connective tissues should be severed with the tips of the scissors.

➤ STEP 5. Undermining of Skin–Muscle Flap

A skin–muscle flap is developed superiorly, laterally, and if necessary, medially, using scissor dissection deep to the orbicularis oculi muscle (see Fig. 5.6). The dissection is carried over the orbital rim, exposing the periosteum.

➤ STEP 6. Periosteal Incision

The skin–muscle flap is retracted exposing the area for surgery. The periosteum is then incised in the middle of the orbital rim with a scalpel (see Fig. 5.7).

➤ STEP 7. Subperiosteal Dissection of Lateral Orbital Rim and Lateral Orbit

Periosteal elevators are used to perform subperiosteal dissection of the orbit and orbital rims (see Fig. 5.8). One must be aware of the lacrimal fossa, a deep concavity in the superolateral orbit. When reflecting the periosteum from the lateral orbital rim into the orbit, the periosteal elevator must be turned so that it extends almost directly laterally inside the orbital rim. If the periosteum is violated, the lacrimal gland may herniate into the surgical field.

This approach affords excellent access to the entire lateral orbital rim, as well as the lateral and superior walls of the internal orbit (see Fig. 5.9).

➤ STEP 8. Closure

The wound is closed in three layers, the periosteum (see Fig. 5.10), the muscle (see Fig. 5.11), and the skin (see Fig. 5.12). It is especially important to close the orbicularis oculi muscle laterally, over the orbital rim, to prevent thinning of the soft tissues covering the bone.

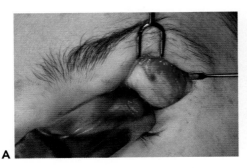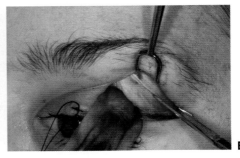

FIGURE 5.7 A: Photograph showing the supraperiosteal exposure of the orbital rim. **B:** An incision is made through the periosteum along the lateral orbital rim.

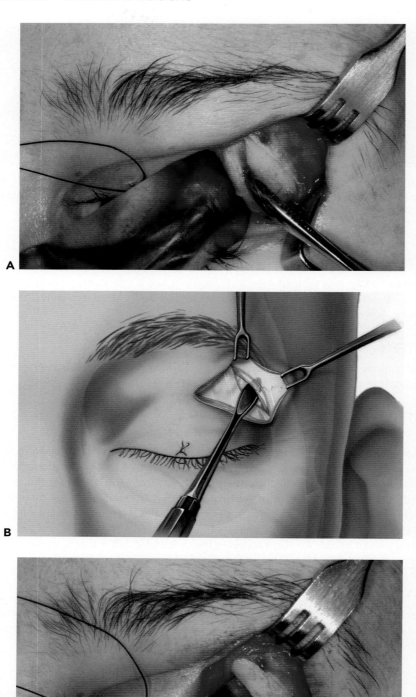

FIGURE 5.8 A: Photograph showing the use of a periosteal elevator to strip the periosteum along the lateral orbital rim. Illustration **(B)** and photograph **(C)** showing dissection inside the orbit. The tip of the periosteal elevator must be kept in contact with the bone as dissection into the orbit proceeds. To facilitate retraction of the skin–muscle flap, it can be widely undermined laterally.

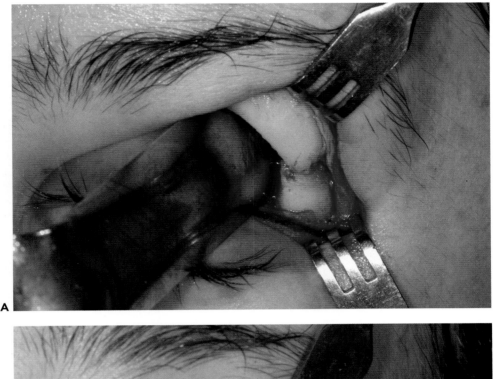

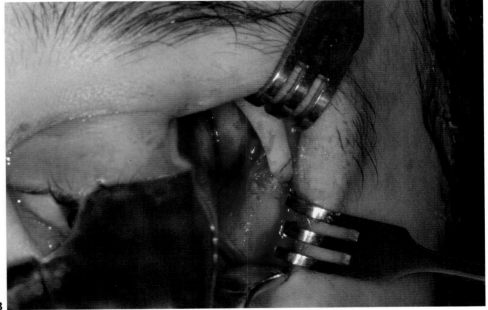

FIGURE 5.9 Photographs showing exposure of lateral orbital rim and frontozygomatic suture **(A)**, as well as the superolateral wall of the internal orbit **(B)**.

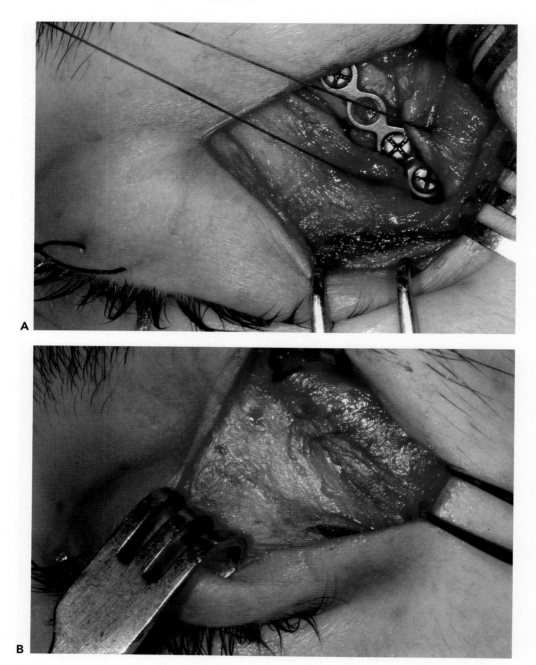

FIGURE 5.10 Photographs showing periosteal closure. A 3-0 polyglactin suture is used to tightly close the periosteum over the top of the lateral orbital rim. Before **(A)** and after **(B)** closure.

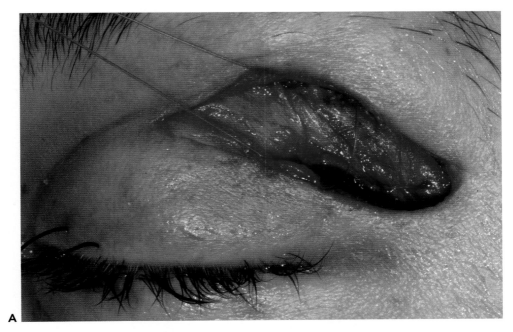

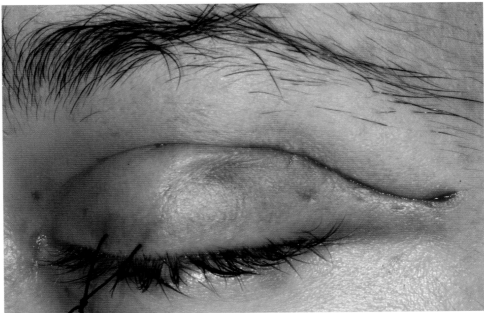

FIGURE 5.11 Photographs showing closure of the orbicularis oculi muscle. A 4-0 chromic catgut suture is placed through the cut edges of the muscle **(A)** to reapproximate it. Once four or five sutures have been placed, the skin edges should appose one another without dehiscence **(B)**.

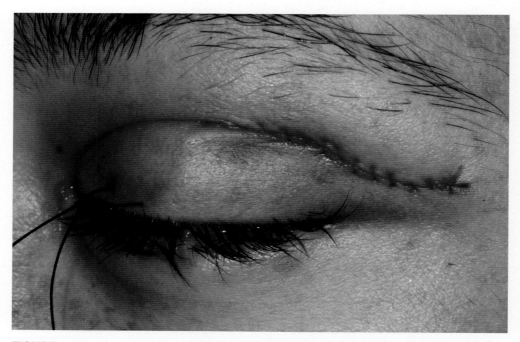

FIGURE 5.12 Photograph showing closure of the skin with running fast-absorbing 6-0 gut suture.

SECTION 3

Coronal Approach

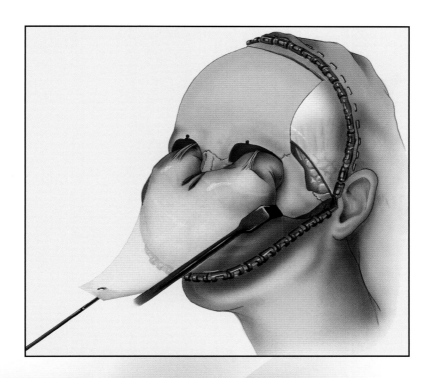

SECTION 3

Coronal Approach

6

Coronal Approach

The coronal or bitemporal incision is a versatile surgical approach to the upper and middle regions of the facial skeleton, including the zygomatic arch. It provides excellent access to these areas with minimal complications (1). A major advantage of this approach is that most of the surgical scar is hidden within the hairline. When the incision is extended into the preauricular area, the surgical scar is inconspicuous.

Surgical Anatomy

Layers of the Scalp

The basic mnemonic for the layers of the scalp (see Fig. 6.1) is "SCALP": S, skin; C, subcutaneous tissue; A, aponeurosis and muscle; L, loose areolar tissue; P, pericranium (periosteum).

The skin and subcutaneous tissue of the scalp are surgically inseparable, unlike these same structures elsewhere in the body. Many hair follicles and sweat glands are found in the subcutaneous fat just beneath the dermis. In addition, no easy plane of cleavage exists between the subcutaneous fat and the musculoaponeurotic layer.

The musculoaponeurotic layer, also inappropriately called the galea (which refers to aponeurosis *only*), consists of the paired frontalis (epicranius) and occipitalis muscles, the auricular muscles, and a broad aponeurosis. The aponeurosis is the true galea and has two portions, an extensive intermediate aponeurosis between the frontalis and occipitalis muscles and a lateral extension into the temporoparietal region, which is known as the *temporoparietal fascia*. Farther inferiorly, the temporoparietal fascia is continuous with the superficial musculoaponeurotic system (SMAS) of the face. The paired frontalis muscles originate from the galeal aponeurosis and insert into the dermis at the level of the eyebrows. An extension of the galea separates the two quadrilateral frontalis muscles in the midline of the forehead.

The galea is a dense, glistening sheet of fibrous tissue, approximately 0.5 mm thick, stretching between the occipitalis and frontalis muscles. When the galea moves, the skin and fat move with it because they are closely attached. Laterally, the galea (or *temporoparietal fascia*, as it is usually called) becomes less dense but is still readily dissectible. The superficial temporal artery lies on or in this layer.

The subgaleal fascia is the layer usually referred to as *the loose areolar layer* or the *subaponeurotic plane*. This layer cleaves readily, allowing the skin, subcutaneous tissue, and musculoaponeurotic layers to be stripped from the pericranium. It is in this fascial plane that cleavage occurs during traumatic avulsion of the scalp. The loose tissue of the subgaleal fascia allows for free movement of the skin over the periosteum when the frontalis muscle is contracted.

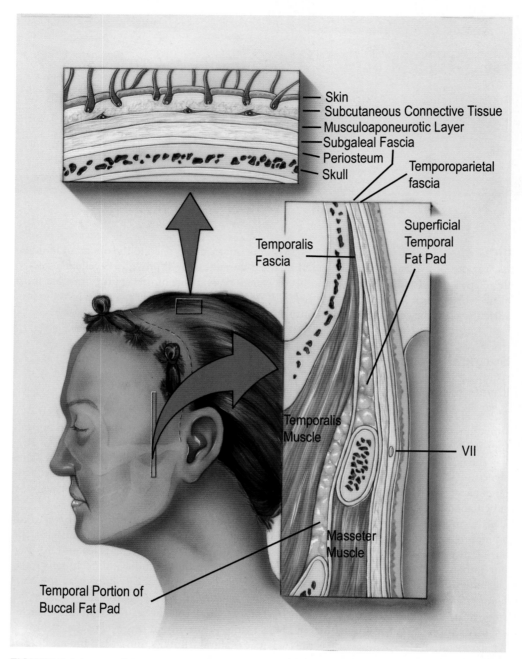

Skin
Subcutaneous Connective Tissue
Musculoaponeurotic Layer
Subgaleal Fascia
Periosteum
Skull

Temporoparietal fascia

Superficial Temporal Fat Pad

Temporalis Fascia

Temporalis Muscle

VII

Masseter Muscle

Temporal Portion of Buccal Fat Pad

FIGURE 6.1 Layers of the scalp above the superior temporal line (***top inset***) and below the superior temporal line (***right inset***). **Top inset:** Skin, subcutaneous tissues, the musculoaponeurotic layer (galea in this illustration), the subgaleal layer of loose tissue, the periosteum (pericranium), and the skull bone. **Right inset:** Skin, subcutaneous tissues, the temporoparietal fascia (note temporal branch of VII nerve), the superficial layer of temporalis fascia, a superficial pad of fat, the deep layer of temporalis fascia, the temporalis muscle above, the buccal fat pad below, and skull.

Anatomic dissections have also revealed that the subgaleal fascia can be mobilized as an independent fascial layer. For the routine coronal approach to the facial skeleton, however, this fascial layer is used only for its ease of cleavage.

Anteriorly, the subgaleal fascia is continuous with the loose areolar layer deep to the orbicularis oculi muscles. Laterally, it is attached to the frontal process of the zygoma. This attachment continues along the superior surface of the zygomatic arch, above the external auditory meatus, and over the mastoid process. It terminates by fusing with the periosteum along the superior nuchal line.

The pericranium is the periosteum of the skull. It can be elevated from the skull, although it is more firmly attached along cranial sutures. When released by subperiosteal dissection, the pericranium retracts owing to its elasticity.

Layers of the Temporoparietal Region

The temporoparietal fascia is the most superficial fascial layer beneath the subcutaneous fat (Fig. 6.1). Frequently called the *superficial temporal fascia* or the *suprazygomatic SMAS*, this fascial layer is the lateral extension of the galea and is continuous with the SMAS of the face (see Fig. 6.2). Because the fascia is just beneath the skin, it may go unrecognized after incision. The blood vessels of the scalp, such as the superficial temporal vessels, run along the outer aspect of the fascia, adjacent to the subcutaneous fat. The motor nerves, such as the temporal branch of the facial nerve, run on its deep surface.

The subgaleal fascia in the temporoparietal region is well developed and can be dissected as a discrete fascial layer, although it is used only as a cleavage plane in the standard coronal approach (Fig. 6.2).

The temporalis fascia is the fascia of the temporalis muscle. This thick layer arises from the superior temporal line, where it fuses with the pericranium (Fig. 6.1). The temporalis muscle arises from the deep surface of the temporalis fascia and the whole of the temporal fossa. At the level of the superior orbital rim, the temporalis fascia splits, with the superficial layer attaching to the lateral border and the deep layer attaching to the medial border of the zygomatic arch. A small quantity of fat, sometimes called the

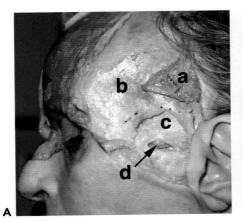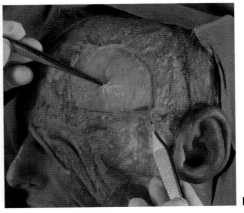

FIGURE 6.2 A: Anatomic dissection of the temporal region showing temporoparietal fascia (*a*), superficial layer of the temporalis fascia (*b*), superficial temporal fat pad (*c*), and temporalis muscle showing through an opening in the deep layer of the temporalis fascia (*d*). Between the temporoparietal fascia (*a*) and the superficial temporalis fascia (*b*) is the subgaleal layer, which is continuous with this same layer in the scalp. **B:** Anatomic dissection of the temporal region showing the temporoparietal fascia (lower forceps) and the subgaleal fascia (upper forceps). Skin and subcutaneous tissues have been removed.

superficial temporal fat pad, separates the two layers. Dissection through the medial layer of the temporalis fascia reveals another layer of fat, the temporal portion of the buccal fat pad, which is continuous with the other portions of the buccal fat pad of the cheek below the zygomatic arch. This fat pad separates the temporalis muscle from the zygomatic arch and from the other muscles of mastication, allowing a smooth gliding motion while functioning.

Temporal Branch of Facial Nerve

The temporal branches of the facial nerve are often called the *frontal branches* when they reach the supraciliary region. The nerves provide motor innervation to the frontalis, to the corrugator, to the procerus, and occasionally, to a portion of the orbicularis oculi muscles. Nerve injury is revealed by the inability to raise the eyebrow or wrinkle the forehead.

The temporal branch or branches of the facial nerve leave the parotid gland immediately inferior to the zygomatic arch (see Fig. 6.3). The general course is from a point 0.5 cm below the tragus to a point 1.5 cm above the lateral eyebrow (2). It crosses superficial to the zygomatic arch at an average distance of 2 cm anterior to the anterior concavity of the external auditory canal, but in some cases it is as near as 0.8 cm or as far as 3.5 cm anterior to the external auditory canal (see Fig. 6.4) (3). As the temporal branch crosses the lateral surface of the arch, it courses along the undersurface of the temporoparietal fascia, between it and the fusion of periosteum of the zygomatic arch, the superficial layer of temporalis fascia, and the

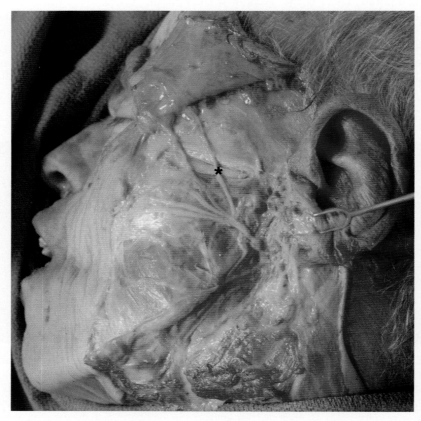

FIGURE 6.3 Anatomic dissection showing branches of the facial nerve. Note the relation of the temporal branch to the zygomatic arch (*). In this specimen, the branch crosses just anterior to the articular eminence of the temporomandibular joint.

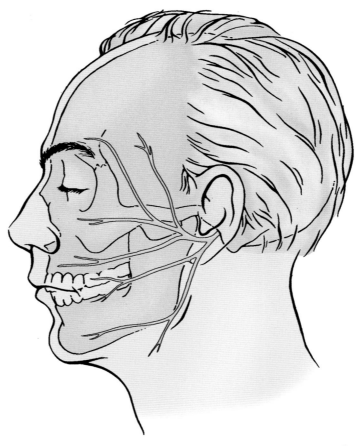

FIGURE 6.4 Branches of the facial nerve. The distance from the anterior concavity of the external auditory canal to the crossing of the zygomatic arch by the temporal branch varies from 8 to 35 mm.

subgaleal fascia (Fig. 6.1). As the nerve courses anterosuperiorly toward the frontalis muscle, it lies on the undersurface of the temporoparietal fascia (see Fig. 6.5) and enters the frontalis muscle no more than 2 cm above the level of the superior orbital rim. It usually branches into three or four rami along its course. The anterior branches supply the superior portion of the orbicularis oculi muscle and the frontalis muscle. The posterior branch innervates the anterior auricular muscles.

The Medial Orbit

The medial orbital wall is composed of several bones: the frontal process of the maxilla, the lacrimal bone, the lamina papyracea of the ethmoid, and part of the lesser wing of the sphenoid. In terms of function, the medial orbit can be divided into anterior, middle, and posterior thirds.

Anterior One Third of the Medial Orbital Wall The medial orbital rim and the anterior one third of the medial orbit comprise the frontal process of the maxilla, the maxillary process of the frontal bone, and the lacrimal bone. The lacrimal fossa for the lacrimal sac lies between the anterior and posterior lacrimal crests. The anterior crest is a continuation of the frontal process of the maxilla. The posterior lacrimal crest is an extension of the lacrimal bone. The bone of the lateral nasal wall contains the nasolacrimal duct, which enters the nasal cavity through the inferior meatus located beneath the inferior turbinate.

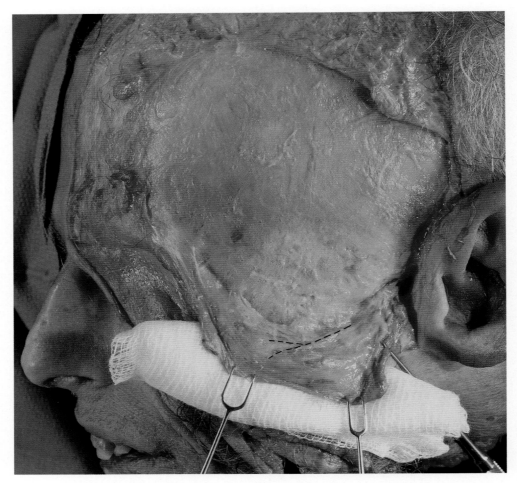

FIGURE 6.5 Anatomic dissection showing the position of the temporal branch of the facial nerve in relation to the temporoparietal fascia and zygomatic arch. The temporoparietal fascia is retracted inferiorly. The temporal branch of the facial nerve courses on its deep surface (or within the layer of fascia) anteriorly and superiorly (*dashed lines*), between the temporoparietal fascia and the point of fusion of the superficial layer of the temporalis fascia with the periosteum of the zygomatic arch.

Middle One Third of the Medial Orbital Wall The middle one third of the medial orbital wall, largely made of the lamina papyracea of the ethmoid bone, is thin, but it is reinforced by the buttress effect of the ethmoid air cells. The only vascular structures of any significance are the anterior and posterior ethmoidal arteries. The foramina for the anterior and posterior ethmoid arteries and nerves are found in, or just above, the frontoethmoid suture line at the level of the cribriform plate. The anterior ethmoid foramen is located approximately 24 mm posterior to the anterior lacrimal crest (4) (see Fig. 6.6). The posterior ethmoid foramen or foramina (25% are multiple) are located approximately 36 mm posterior to the anterior lacrimal crest (4). The optic canal is located approximately 42 mm posterior to the anterior lacrimal crest. The distance between the posterior ethmoidal artery and the optic nerve is variable, but it is never less than 3 mm (4).

Posterior One Third of the Medial Orbital Wall The posterior part of the orbit is made of thick bone surrounding the optic foramen and superior orbital fissure.

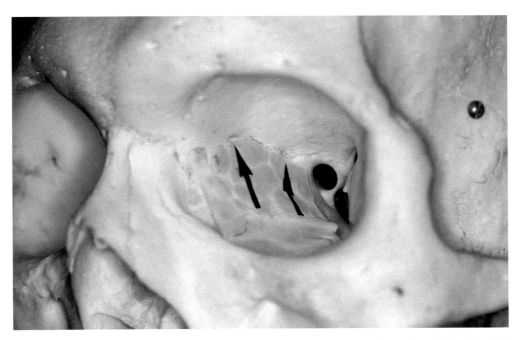

FIGURE 6.6 Medial orbital wall of the skull. Note the position of the anterior and posterior ethmoidal foramina. They are not located at the most superior portion of the orbit but at the level of the cribriform plate.

Technique

The coronal approach can be used to expose different areas of the upper and middle face (Video 6.1). The layer of dissection and the extent of exposure depend on the particular surgical procedure for which the coronal approach is used. In some instances, it may be prudent to perform a subperiosteal elevation of the coronal flap from the point of incision. The periosteum is freed with a scalpel along the superior temporal lines as one proceeds anteriorly with the dissection, leaving the temporalis muscles attached to the skull. In most cases, however, dissection and elevation of the coronal flap are in the easily cleavable subgaleal plane. The deeper pericranium may be used as a separate vascularized coronal flap for defect coverage. For illustrative purposes, the following description of the complete exposure of the upper and middle face, including the zygomatic arch, using a subgaleal dissection for most of the flap elevation is given.

➤ **STEP 1.** Locating the Incision Line and Preparation

Two factors are considered when designing the line of incision. The first is the hairline of the patient. In men, hairline recession at the widow's peak and the lateral temporal valleys should be considered. For balding men, the incision might be placed along a line extending from one preauricular area to the other, several centimeters behind the hairline (see Fig. 6.7), or even more posteriorly. Incisions made further posteriorly need not reduce access to the operative field because the extent of skeletal exposure depends on the inferior extent of the incisions and not on the anteroposterior position. In men who are not balding and in most women, the incision may be curved anteriorly at the vertex, paralleling but remaining 4 to 5 cm within the hairline (see Fig. 6.8). In children, the incision is preferably placed well behind the hairline to allow for migration of the scar with growth. In black patients with short hair, keloid formation is also a concern. Zigzag incisions may be used to make the scars less noticeable. If a hemicoronal incision is planned, the incision curves forward at the midline, ending just posterior to the hairline. Curving the hemicoronal incision anteriorly provides the relaxation necessary for the retraction of the flap.

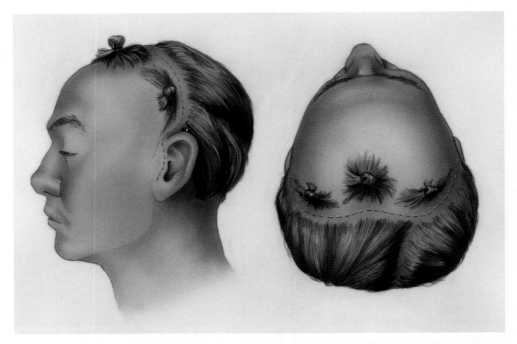

FIGURE 6.7 Incision placement for patients with male pattern hair recession. The incision is stepped posteriorly just above the attachment of the helix of the ear. The incision can be moved more posteriorly as necessary.

The second factor considered while designing the location of the incision is the extent of inferior access required for the procedure. When exposure of the zygomatic arch is unnecessary, extending the coronal incision inferiorly to the level of the helix may be all that is necessary. However, the coronal incision can be extended inferiorly to the level of the earlobe as a preauricular incision. This maneuver allows exposure of the zygomatic arch, temporomandibular joint (TMJ), and/or infraorbital rims.

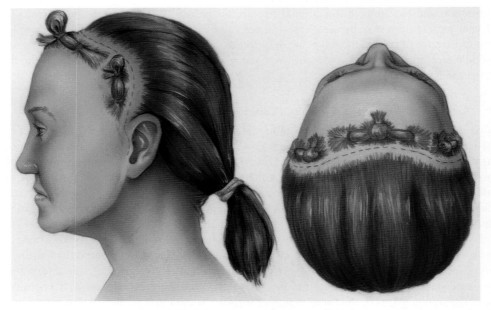

FIGURE 6.8 Incision placement for most female patients and for those male patients with no signs or family history of baldness. The incision is kept approximately 4 cm behind the hairline.

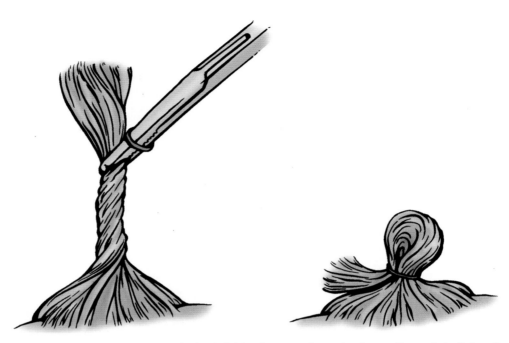

FIGURE 6.9 The technique of gathering hair into clumps and securing them with small elastic bands. Small bundles of hair are twisted with fingers and each bundle is grasped in the middle with a hemostat loaded with an elastic band. The elastic band is rolled off the hemostat onto the hair bundle below the tips of the hemostat, which can be removed.

Shaving of the head before incision is not medically necessary for sterility and should be customized for surgical exposure and the patient's preferences. In fact, the presence of hair helps to determine the direction of the hair shafts and may guide incision level to minimize damage to the follicles. The presence of hair makes closure more difficult, but it does not seem to cause an increase in the rate of infection. A comb can be used to separate the hair along the proposed incision line. Long hair can be held in clumps, with elastics placed either before or after sterile preparation. This measure minimizes the annoyance caused by loose hair in the surgical field (see Fig. 6.9). If shaving of the head is required, it need not be extensive; a small strip, approximately 12 to 15 mm, is adequate. The drapes can be sutured or stapled to the scalp approximately 1.5 cm posterior to the planned incision site, covering the posterior scalp and confining the hair.

➤ **STEP 2.** Hemostatic Techniques

Blood loss from the coronal incision is greatest at the beginning and end of the surgery. Three techniques may be used to reduce blood loss. In the first technique, a vasoconstrictor is injected into the subgaleal plane to promote hemostasis and to help separate the tissue layers. The second technique involves inserting running blocking sutures of 2-0 polypropylene or nylon along each side of the proposed incision line. These sutures are removed at the completion of scalp closure. In the last technique, special cautery scalpels are used for scalp incisions, but these heated scalpels may damage hair follicles. Multiple measures may be useful for those individuals such as pediatric patients in whom blood loss must be kept to an absolute minimum.

➤ **STEP 3.** Incision

Crosshatches, scratches, or tattoo dye markings across the proposed site of incision assist in properly aligning the scalp during closure. The first marking is made in the midline and subsequent marks are made laterally at approximately equal distances from the midline (see Fig. 6.10). Crosshatches made with a scalpel tip should be deep enough (until bleeding) so that their location is visible at the end of the surgical procedure.

The initial portion of the incision is made with a no. 10 blade or a special diathermy knife, extending from one superior temporal line to the other. For routine coronal exposure, the

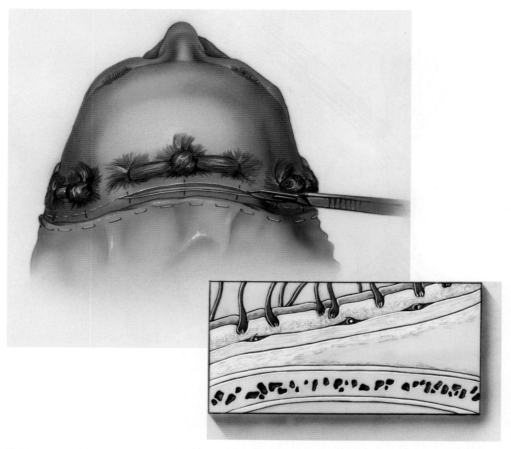

FIGURE 6.10 Draping of the patient and the initial incision. The drapes are secured with staples and/or sutures just posterior to the location of the planned incision. Crosshatches are scored into the scalp at several locations for realignment of the flap during closure. The initial incision extends from one superior temporal line to the other, to the depth of the pericranium (***inset***). The dissection will be in the subgaleal plane, which is loose connective tissue and cleaves readily.

incision is through the skin, subcutaneous tissue, and galea (Fig. 6.10), revealing the subgaleal plane of loose areolar connective tissue overlying the pericranium. The flap margin may be rapidly and easily lifted and dissected above the pericranium. Limiting the initial incision to the area between the two superior temporal lines prevents incising through the temporalis fascia into the temporalis musculature, which bleeds freely.

The skin incision below the superior temporal line should extend to the depth of the glistening superficial layer of the temporalis fascia, into the subgaleal plane, continuous with the dissection above the superior temporal line. An easy method to ensure that the incision is made to the proper depth is to bluntly dissect in the subgaleal plane from above, toward the zygomatic arch, with curved scissors and to incise to that depth (see Fig. 6.11).

Preauricular extension of the incision is made within a preauricular skin fold to the level of the lobule. The dissection severs the preauricular muscle and follows the cartilaginous external auditory canal (refer to the dissection described in Chapter 12).

➤ **STEP 4.** Elevation of the Coronal Flap and Exposure of the Zygomatic Arch

After elevation of the anterior and posterior wound margins by 1 to 2 cm, hemostatic clips (Raney clips) may be applied or bleeding vessels isolated and cauterized. Indiscriminate cauterization of the edge of the incised scalp produces alopecia and should be avoided. Some surgeons place an unfolded gauze sponge over the cut edge of the scalp before clip application.

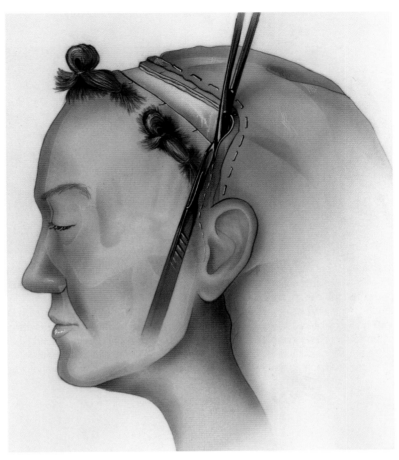

FIGURE 6.11 One technique for incising the scalp in the temporal region. Scissor dissection of the scalp in the subgaleal plane can proceed inferiorly from the previous incision made above the superior temporal line. While the scissors are spread, a scalpel incises to them, preventing the surgeon from incising the temporalis fascia and muscle, which bleed freely.

The gauze can be pulled off the scalp prior to closure, after removing the accompanying row of clips. In some instances, bleeding is encountered during the procedure from small emissary veins exiting through the pericranium or exposed skull. Cauterization, bone wax application, or both are useful in such instances.

The flap may be elevated atop the pericranium with finger dissection, with blunt periosteal elevators or by back cutting with a scalpel (or electrocautery) (see Fig. 6.12). As dissection proceeds anteriorly, tension develops because the flap is still attached laterally over the temporalis muscles. Dissecting that portion of the flap below the superior temporal line from the temporalis fascia relieves this tension and allows the flap to retract further anteriorly. Along the lateral aspect of the skull, the glistening white temporalis fascia becomes visible where it blends with the pericranium at the superior temporal line. The plane of dissection is just superficial to this thick fascial sheet.

Once the flap has been dissected anteriorly and inferiorly several centimeters, it should be possible to evert the flap so that the galeal surface is superficial (see Fig. 6.13). If it is not possible to evert the flap, more dissection inferiorly along the superficial layer of the temporalis fascia, and possibly extending the skin incision more inferiorly, may be necessary.

Depending upon the operative procedure, two methods of periosteal incisions can be performed to expose the facial skeleton. For most procedures on the midface, dissection of the flap continues anteriorly in the subgaleal fascial plane until a point 3 to 4 cm superior to the supraorbital rims. A finger is used to palpate and locate the superior temporal lines, and a horizontal incision is made through the pericranium from one superior temporal line to the

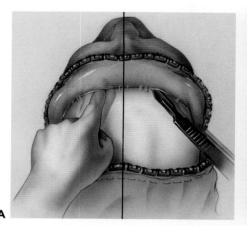
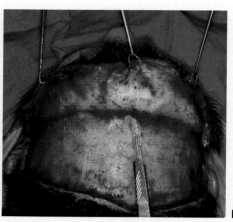

FIGURE 6.12 A: Illustration showing two methods of dissecting the flap in the subgaleal plane. **Left:** Finger dissection readily cleaves the areolar tissue in the subgaleal plane. Several centimeters above the orbital rims, however, the pericranium is more tightly bound to the frontalis muscle and the periosteum may strip from the bone while using this technique in this location. **Right** and photograph **B:** Dissection with a scalpel. The flap is lifted gently with retractors and/or hooks to maintain gentle tension. The back (dull) edge of the scalpel rests on the pericranium and is swept back and forth, allowing the point of the scalpel to incise the subgaleal tissue. This technique is especially useful in those flaps elevated for a second or third time, in which adhesions in the subgaleal layer are more common and must be sharply incised.

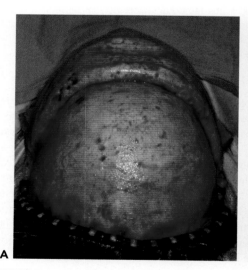
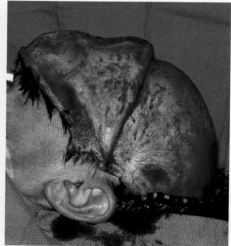

FIGURE 6.13 Photographs showing the coronal flap once it has been dissected to within 3 to 4 cm of the supraorbital rims. **A:** Superior and **(B)** lateral views. Notice that the flap is free enough to passively remain inverted.

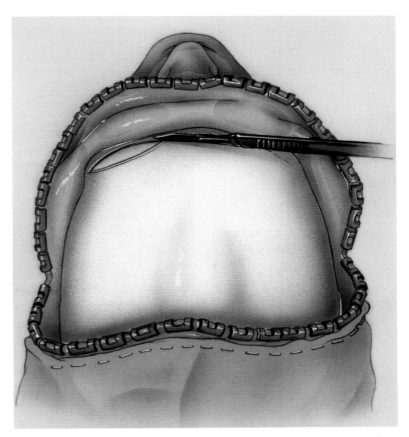

FIGURE 6.14 Incision of periosteum across the forehead from one superior temporal line to the other. The incision through the periosteum should be 3 to 4 cm superior to the orbital rims.

other (see Fig. 6.14). The incision should not be extended beyond the superior temporal line or the temporalis muscle will be cut and begin to bleed. The subperiosteal dissection then continues to the supraorbital rims.

When procedures are performed on the frontal sinus and/or anterior cranial base, it is prudent to develop a vascularized pericranial flap. This flap can be used to fill defects or the frontal sinus, to partition the nose from the sinus or anterior cranial fossa, and so on. The development of a pericranial flap is simple and should be used routinely in coronal approaches to the facial skeleton for trauma repairs. To develop the flap, it is easiest to perform a supraperiosteal dissection, as discussed earlier, and then to elevate the pericranium from the skull. Incisions through the pericranium are made just above the superior temporal lines, extending from the superior orbital rims bilaterally to the posterior extent of the coronal incision (see Fig. 6.15A). An incision is then made through the pericranium from one superior temporal line to the other in the coronal plane, extending to the other incisions through the pericranium (Fig. 6.15B). Periosteal elevators are then used to elevate the pericranium, taking care to avoid tearing the tissue (Fig. 6.15C). Once the pericranium is elevated, the extensive pericranial flap provides a large apron of vascularized tissue for possible use during the surgical procedure (Fig. 6.15D).

No matter which of these techniques is used to incise the pericranium, the dissection is continued in the subperiosteal plane anteriorly to the superior orbital rims.

The lateral portion of the flap is dissected inferiorly atop the temporalis fascia. Once the lateral portion of the flap has been elevated to within 2 to 4 cm of the body of the zygoma and zygomatic arch, these structures can usually be palpated through the covering fascia. Near the ear, the flap is dissected inferiorly to the root of the zygomatic arch. The *superficial layer of temporalis fascia* is incised at the root of the zygomatic arch, just in front of the ear,

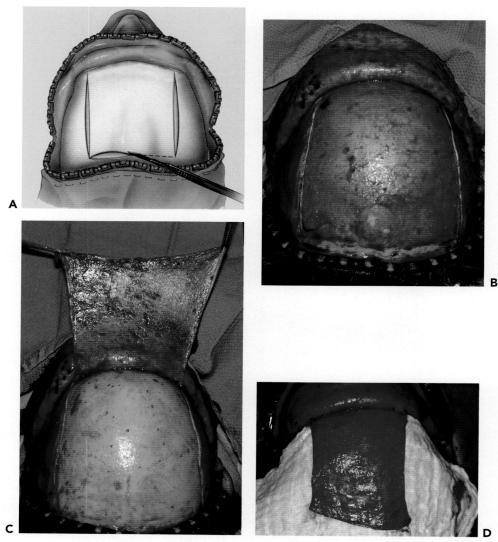

FIGURE 6.15 A: Illustration showing the incisions for development of a pericranial flap. Photographs showing incisions through the pericranium **(B)**, pericranial flap after elevation **(C)**, and pericranial flap lying *in situ* **(D)** demonstrating vasculature.

and the incision is continued anteriorly and superiorly at a 45-degree angle, joining the cross-forehead incision previously made through the pericranium at the superior temporal line (see Fig. 6.16A and B). Incision of the superficial layer of temporalis fascia reveals fat and areolar tissue (Fig. 6.16C and D). The layer of fat should be left undisturbed as far as possible to prevent "temporal hollowing," which occurs when fat settles inferiorly. Dissection made inferiorly should be just deep to the superficial layer of the temporalis fascia, stripping it from the underlying fat. This layer provides a safe route of access to the zygomatic arch because the temporal branch of the facial nerve is always lateral to the superficial layer of the temporalis fascia (see Fig. 6.17A and B). Metzenbaum scissors are used to bluntly dissect just under the superficial layer of the temporalis fascia (Fig. 6.15C). Once the superior surface of the zygomatic arch and the posterior border of the body of the zygoma are

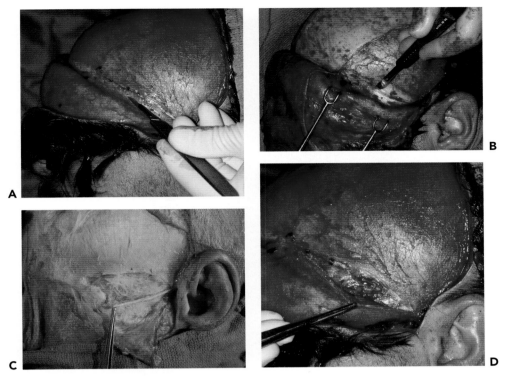

FIGURE 6.16 Incision through the superficial layer of the temporalis fascia. The incision begins at the root of the zygomatic arch (above the temporomandibular joint) upward and forward toward the superior orbital rim. Photographs demonstrating the incision through the superficial layer of the temporalis fascia in a patient who had an incision made through the pericranium just above the orbital rims **(A)** and a patient who had a pericranial flap developed **(B)**. Note the underlying fat between this layer of fascia and the deep layer of the temporalis fascia in a cadaveric dissection **(C)** and in a patient **(D)**. The temporoparietal fascia with the temporal branch of the facial nerve is folded inferiorly (below).

palpable or visible, an incision is made through the periosteum along their superior surface. The incision is continued superiorly along the posterior border of the body of the zygoma and the orbital rim, ultimately meeting the cross-forehead horizontal incision through the pericranium or the area where the pericranial flap has been elevated. Subperiosteal elevation exposes the lateral surfaces of the zygomatic arch, the body of the zygoma, and the lateral orbital rim (see Fig. 6.18).

➤ **STEP 5.** Subperiosteal Exposure of the Periorbital Areas

To allow functional access to the superior orbits and/or nasal region, it is necessary to release the supraorbital neurovascular bundle from its notch or foramen. This maneuver involves dissecting in the subperiosteal plane completely around the bundle, including inside the orbit. If no bone is noted inferior to the bundle, the bundle can be gently removed from the bony notch. However if a foramen is found, a small osteotome can be used to remove the bony bridge along the supraorbital rim to release the bundle (see Fig. 6.19).

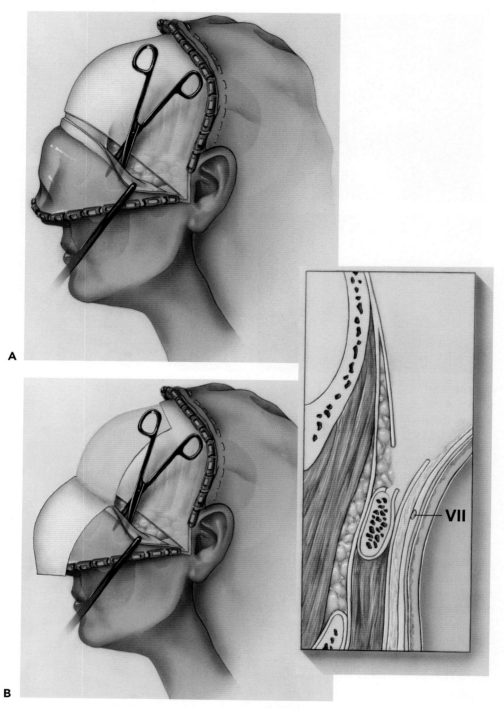

FIGURE 6.17 One method to approach the posterior portion of the lateral orbital rim and the superior surface of the zygomatic arch is demonstrated in these illustrations. **A:** Illustration of patients whose incision through the pericranium is just above the orbital rims and **(B)** in patients who develop a pericranial flap. Dissection with scissors continues deep to the superficial layer of temporalis fascia (***inset***), within the superficial temporal fat pad, until bone is encountered **(C)**. A sharp incision is then made through the periosteum on the superior surface of the zygomatic arch and the posterior surface of the zygoma.

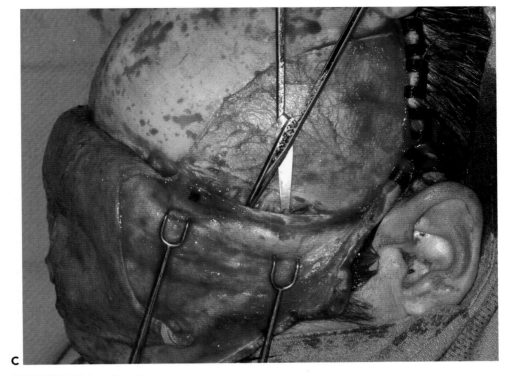

C

FIGURE 6.17 (*continued*)

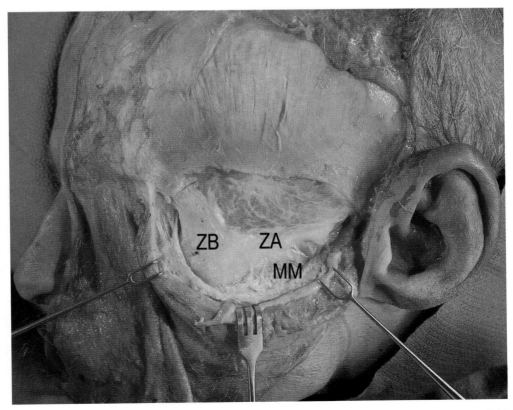

FIGURE 6.18 Anatomic dissection showing the zygomatic arch (*ZA*) and body (*ZB*). The superficial layer of the temporalis fascia and the periosteum is retracted inferiorly and anteriorly. Note the masseter muscle (*MM*) attachment to the inferior portion of the zygomatic arch.

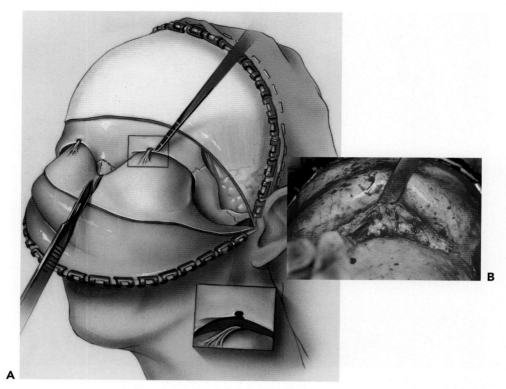

FIGURE 6.19 A: Illustration showing two key features: removal of the bone inferior to the supraorbital foramen (when present) so that the neurovascular bundle can be released and placement of relaxing incisions in the sagittal plane through the elevated periosteum over the bridge of the nose. The use of this technique **(B)** facilitates dissection more inferiorly along the nasal dorsum.

Further retraction of the flap inferiorly may be accomplished by subperiosteal dissection into the orbits. The orbital contents attached to the lateral orbital tubercle are stripped, allowing dissection deep into the lateral orbit. Release of the periosteum around the inferior rim of the orbit allows exposure of the entire orbital floor and infraorbital region. Access to the infraorbital area is easiest after overlying tissues of the zygomatic arch and body are released to relax the overlying envelope.

Dissecting the periosteum from the superior and medial orbital walls releases the flap and allows retraction down to the level of the junction of the nasal bones and upper lateral nasal cartilages. This technique is facilitated by carefully incising the periosteum of the nasofrontal region (Fig. 6.19). Dissection can proceed along the dorsum to the nasal tip, if necessary (see Fig. 6.20).

The medial canthal tendons should not be inadvertently stripped from the posterior and anterior lacrimal crests. They are identified as dense fibrous attachments in the nasolacrimal fossa (see Fig. 6.21). The entire medial orbital wall may be exposed without stripping the canthal tendons. As subperiosteal dissection is extended posteriorly along the medial orbital wall, the surgeon should be on the lookout for the anterior (and posterior) ethmoidal artery. A simple method to identify and cauterize the artery is to strip the periosteum along the roof of the orbit and inferior to the point where the artery pierces the medial orbital wall. With a periosteal elevator on each side of the foramen, retraction allows the periosteum attached

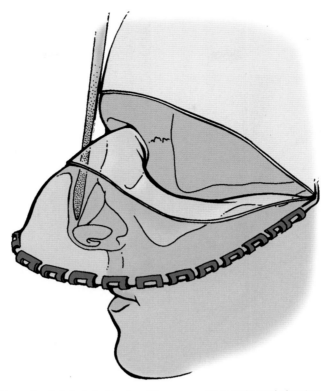

FIGURE 6.20 Dissection inferiorly to the tip of the nose with a periosteal elevator.

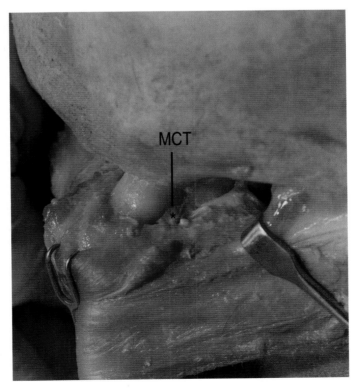

FIGURE 6.21 Anatomic dissection showing the posterior limb of the medial canthal tendon (*MCT*) of the left orbit.

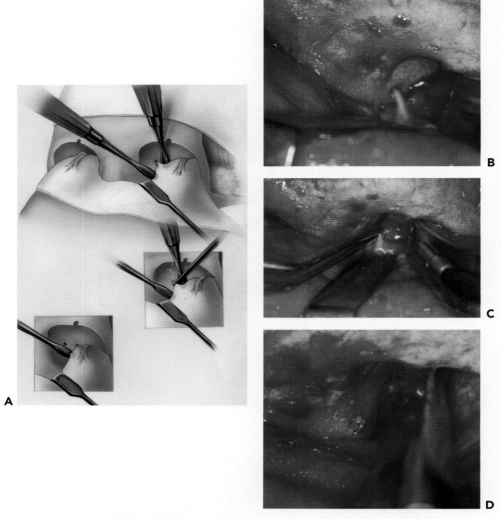

FIGURE 6.22 Dissection of the medial orbital wall. Illustration **(A)** and photographs **(B–D)** showing the sequence of steps necessary to isolate and sever the anterior ethmoidal neurovascular bundle as it exits the medial orbital wall. Periosteal elevators are placed above and below the anterior ethmoidal neurovascular bundle, allowing bipolar cauterization and sectioning.

to the foramen to "tent" outward (see Fig. 6.22). Bipolar cauterization of the artery may be performed, followed by transection. Dissection can then be performed posteriorly by subperiosteal elevation.

After the dissections just described, the upper and middle facial regions are completely exposed (see Fig. 6.23). The entire orbit is dissected from the orbital rims to the apex; the only remaining structure is the medial canthal tendon, unless it was intentionally or inadvertently stripped.

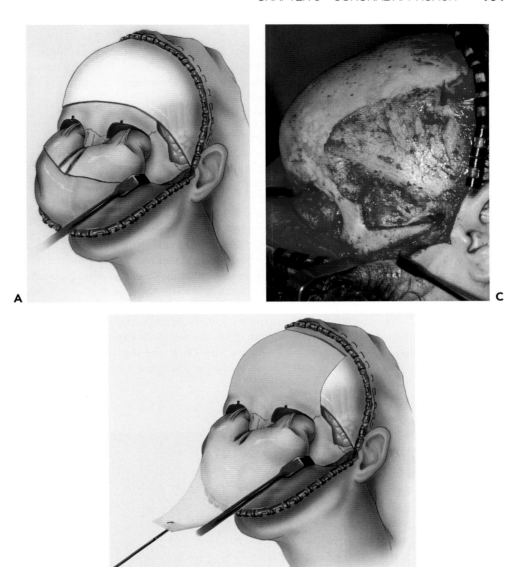

FIGURE 6.23 Amount of exposure obtained with complete dissection of the upper and middle facial bones using the coronal approach. **A:** Illustration in which the pericranial incision was placed just above the orbits. **B:** Illustration in which pericranial flap was elevated (hook). Note the maintenance of attachment of the medial canthal tendon. The infraorbital areas are also exposed if retraction is performed from the side of the orbit. **C:** Photograph showing the exposure after coronal approach using pericranial flap elevation.

➤ **STEP 6.** Exposure of the Temporal Fossa

Access into the temporal fossa is gained by stripping the anterior edge of the temporalis muscle from the temporal surfaces of the zygomatic, temporal, and frontal bones. The entire temporalis muscle is stripped subperiosteally from the temporal fossa if necessary, but care should be taken to preserve the blood supply to the temporalis muscle.

➤ **STEP 7.** Exposure of the Temporomandibular Joint and/or Mandibular Condyle/Ramus

Access to the TMJ region is gained by dissecting below the zygomatic arch (refer to Chapter 12). Exposure of the lateral surface of the mandibular subcondylar region and ramus may commence lateral to the capsule of the TMJ. An incision through the periosteum just inferior to the insertion of the TMJ capsule at the condylar neck will expose the neck of the condyle.

Wider access below the zygomatic arch can be achieved by two maneuvers. In the first approach, the masseter muscle is cut or released from its origin along the zygomatic arch and body, and then stripped from the lateral surface of the mandibular ramus to expose the ramus of the mandible (see Fig. 6.24). The temporalis muscle at the depth of this dissection can be noted as it inserts into the coronoid process. Another approach is to perform an osteotomy of the zygomatic arch, leaving it pedicled to the masseter muscle, and to dissect between the masseter and temporalis muscles, stripping the masseter from the lateral surface of the mandibular ramus. One anatomic consideration is valid with either of these wide-exposure methods: the vascular and neural supply to the masseter muscle courses from the medial side of the mandible through the sigmoid notch into the masseter muscle. Therefore, stripping the masseter from above may severely affect its function.

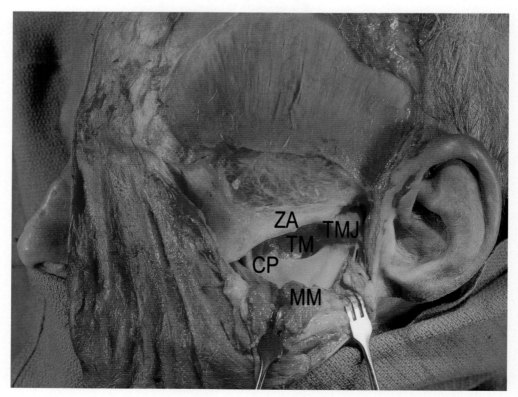

FIGURE 6.24 Anatomic dissection showing exposure of the superior portion of the mandibular ramus through the coronal approach. In this dissection, the masseter muscle (*MM*) is stripped from its origin along the undersurface of the zygomatic arch (*ZA*). The facial nerve is retracted inferiorly and anteriorly. Note the temporomandibular joint capsule (*TMJ*), which has not been entered. The temporalis muscle (*TM*) is still attached to the coronoid process (*CP*) and the medial surface of the mandible.

➤ **STEP 8.** Harvesting Cranial Bone Grafts

One of the many advantages of the coronal approach is that cranial bone graft harvesting is facilitated. If the incision through the pericranium is made just above the orbits, another peri-osteal incision in the region of the parietal bulge allows exposure for harvesting a bone graft (see Fig. 6.25A and B). Closure of the periosteum in such cases precedes scalp closure. In the case where a pericranial flap has been elevated, bone grafts are harvested directly from the exposed cranium (Fig. 6.25C and D) after subperiosteal dissection posteriorly from the point of the original coronal incision.

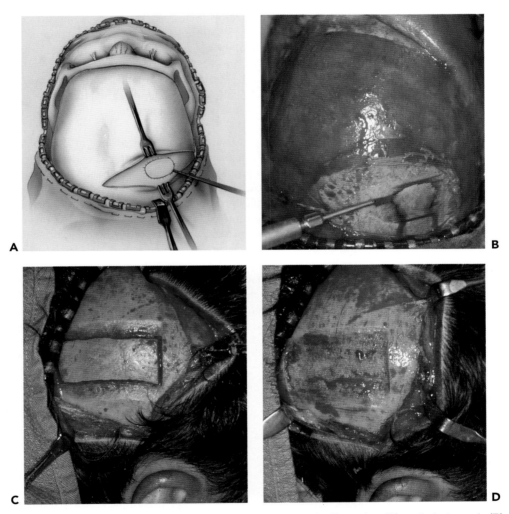

FIGURE 6.25 Bone graft harvest using the coronal approach. Illustration **(A)** and photograph **(B)** showing harvesting of a graft when the pericranial incision is just above the orbital rims. When a peric-ranial approach has been used, the bone can be procured directly **(C, D)**.

➤ **STEP 9.** Closure

Closed suction drainage may be employed by using a flat drain exiting the hair-bearing region of the scalp posterior to the incision. Proper approximation of the sagging, detached tissues recreates optimal esthetic results by minimizing tissue drooping. After wide exposure of the malar and infraorbital regions, suture resuspension of the soft tissues is advocated. Slowly resorbing or permanent 3-0 sutures passed through the deep surface of the periosteum of the malar region are pexed to the temporalis fascia or another stable structure. A lateral canthopexy is also recommended if the canthal attachments to the lateral orbital tubercle are stripped from the bone. Toothed forceps are used to identify the superficial portion of the lateral canthal tendon within the deep surface of the coronal flap. One slowly resorbing or permanent 3-0 suture is placed through the lateral canthus from the deep surface of the coronal flap. The location of the proper vertical position of the canthal tendon can be determined by drawing the suture upward or downward, while observing the configuration of the palpebral fissure. A secure lateral canthopexy of the deep portion of the lateral canthal tendon may be performed by drilling a large hole through the lateral orbital rim just below the frontozygomatic suture. The suture and tendon are then pulled into this hole. However, if anatomic structures have not been disrupted, suitable canthopexy may be accomplished by suturing through the anterior portion of the lateral canthal tendon around the front of the lateral orbital rim, and securing it to a bone screw, a hole in the bone, or the temporalis fascia.

Whenever the temporalis muscle is stripped from the temporal surface of the orbit, it should also be suspended to prevent a hollow appearance in the temporal region. An easy method involves drilling holes through the posterior edge of the orbital rim and suturing the anterior edge of the temporalis muscle with slowly resorbing 3-0 sutures.

Closure of the periosteum around the lateral orbital rim is performed with resorbable 4-0 sutures. Ideally, the periosteum over the zygomatic arch should be closed, but this can be difficult owing to the small amount of periosteum available. Suturing the periosteum may also injure the temporal branch of the facial nerve, which is just superficial to the periosteum. Instead, *oversuspension* of the superficial layer of the temporalis fascia is performed. The inferior edge of the superficial layer of the temporalis fascia, which is incised during the approach, is sutured approximately 1 cm superior to the superior edge of the incised fascia (see Fig. 6.26). Running horizontal, slowly resorbing 3-0 sutures are used for this purpose. Therefore, the tissues lateral to the zygomatic arch are suspended tightly

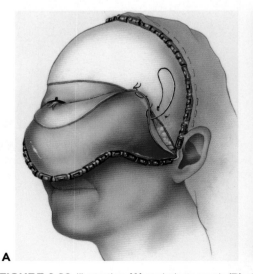
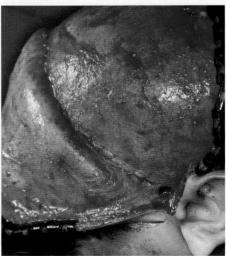

A **B**

FIGURE 6.26 Illustration **(A)** and photograph **(B)** showing suturing of the superficial layer of the temporalis fascia. Note that the inferior edge of fascia is sutured in a more superior location than the cut superior edge.

in a location that is more superior than had the incised superficial temporalis fascia been simply sutured.

It is not necessary to close the horizontal periosteal incision across the forehead. The periosteum in this area is thin and does not hold sutures. Closure of the coronal incision will bring the periosteal tissues into acceptable approximation.

The scalp incision is closed in two layers using slowly resorbing 2-0 sutures through the galea/subcutaneous tissues and resorbing or permanent 2-0 skin sutures (smaller sutures are used in children), or staples. As noted previously, the use of a suction drain (usually 7-mm flat) is optional. The skin sutures/staples are removed in 7 to 10 days.

The preauricular component of the coronal approach should be closed in layers, as in any other preauricular approach.

Pressure dressings are optional, but if used, they should not be tight. Periorbital edema increases greatly with tight pressure dressings on the scalp after coronal approaches.

Alternate Incisions

The coronal incision has been modified repeatedly by surgeons. The principal difference in these surgical techniques involves the position of the skin incision. A major modification has been the placement of the incision behind the ear (see Fig. 6.27) (5,6). The advantage of this

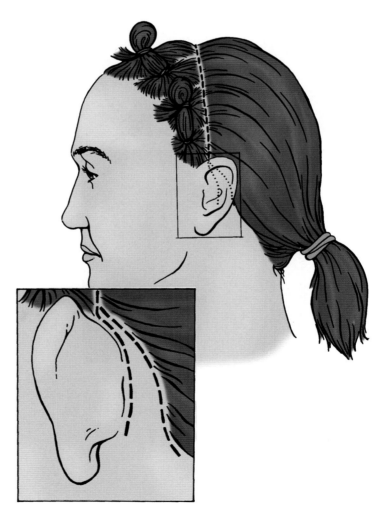

FIGURE 6.27 Postauricular placement of the coronal incision. The incision can be extended into the postauricular sulcus or within the hairline (***inset***).

positioning is further camouflage of the scar. Any inferior extension of the coronal incision can be hidden within the postauricular fold or along the hairline.

Even with well-placed incisions, the scar that forms may produce a separation of the hair that can become visible when the hair is wet, such as during swimming. A modification of the incision has been the use of a zigzag incision instead of a straight incision within the hairline (see Fig. 6.28A and B) (7). The zigzag incision helps to break up the scar and make it less noticeable, even when the hair is worn short (Fig. 6.28C). The major disadvantage of this incision is the increased time needed for closure.

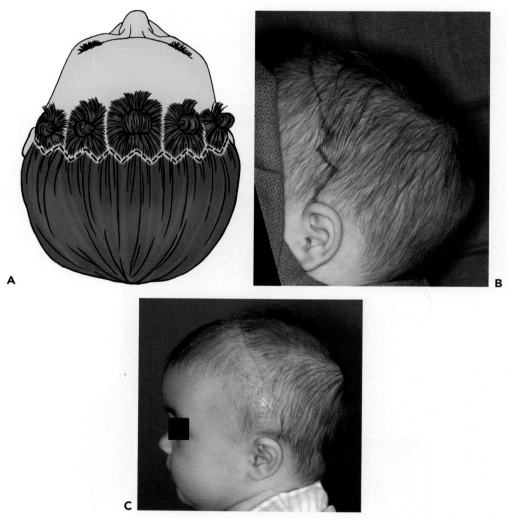

A

B

C

FIGURE 6.28 Zigzag incision to make the scar less obvious. **A:** Illustration showing zigzag incision across the entire incision. Alternatively, the zigzag can be used in the temporal areas only, with a straight incision across the vertex **(B)**. The resultant scar becomes less noticeable **(C)**.

References

1. Shepherd DE, Ward-Booth RP, Moos KF. The morbidity of bicoronal flaps in maxillofacial surgery. *Br J Oral Max Surg.* 1985;23:1.
2. Furnas DW. Landmarks for the trunk and the temporofacial division of the facial nerve. *Br J Surg.* 1965;52:694.
3. Al-Kayat A, Bramley P. A modified pre-auricular approach to the temporomandibular joint and malar arch. *Br J Oral Surg.* 1979;17:91.
4. Rontal E, Rontal M, Guilford FT. Surgical anatomy of the orbit. *Ann Oto Rhinol Laryn* 1979;88:382–386.
5. Polley JW, Cohen M. The retroauricular coronal incision. *Scand J Plast Reconstr Hand Surg.* 1992;26:79.
6. Posnick JC, Goldstein JA, Clokie C. Advantages of the postauricular coronal incision. *Ann Plast Surg.* 1992;29:114.
7. Munro IR, Fearon JA. The coronal incision revisited. *Plast Reconstr Surg.* 1994;93:185.

SECTION 4

Transoral Approaches to the Facial Skeleton

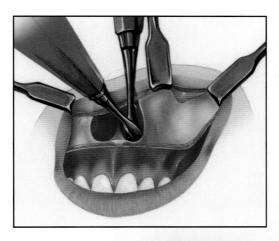 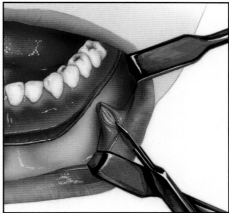

The midfacial and mandibular skeleton can be readily exposed through incisions placed inside the oral cavity. The approaches are rapid and safe and the exposure is excellent. The greatest advantage of such approaches is the hidden scar. This section includes descriptions of the maxillary and mandibular vestibular approaches to the facial skeleton. In addition, two variations of the vestibular approach for maxillary exposure will be presented. The first variation is the midface degloving approach, which, in addition to a vestibular incision, includes intranasal incisions to provide even more access to the maxilla and midface. The second variation is the Weber-Fergusson approach, which combines the vestibular approach with transcutaneous incisions to provide unimpeded access to the maxilla, zygoma, and posterior portions of the midface.

7 Approaches to the Maxilla

The maxilla can be approached through a variety of incisions, but most of it can be exposed with an incision hidden within the oral cavity. The *maxillary vestibular approach* is one of the most useful when performing any of a wide variety of procedures in the midface. It allows relatively safe access to the entire facial surface of the midfacial skeleton, from the zygomatic arch to the infraorbital rim and the frontal process of the maxilla. The greatest advantage of the approach is the hidden intraoral scar that results. The approach is also relatively rapid and simple, and the complications are few. Damage to branches of the facial nerve is nonexistent as long as one stays within the subperiosteal plane, and damage to the infraorbital nerve is rare with proper use of the technique.

When additional exposure is required, the maxillary vestibular approach can be combined with other approaches to broaden the access. Two such approaches, the *facial degloving* and the *Weber-Ferguson*, will be described later.

Surgical Anatomy

Infraorbital Nerve

The only important neurovascular structure that must be negotiated during procedures in the midfacial region is the infraorbital neurovascular bundle. The infraorbital nerve is the largest cutaneous branch of the maxillary division of the trigeminal nerve. The artery and vein that accompany the infraorbital nerve are surgically insignificant. The nerve exits the infraorbital foramen, 7 to 10 mm inferior to the infraorbital rim just medial to the zygomaticomaxillary suture, or approximately at the medial and middle thirds of the orbit. After exiting the infraorbital foramen, the infraorbital nerve divides into terminal branches that spread fanlike into the lower eyelid, nose, and upper lip. The palpebral branches turn upward to supply the lower eyelid; the nasal branches supply the skin on the lateral surface of the lower half of the nose. Three of the four superior labial branches enter the lip between its muscles and the mucous membrane. These nerves supply not only the mucous membrane of the upper lip, but also its skin, which they reach by perforating the orbicularis oris muscle. Damage to this nerve results in loss of sensation in these areas, and possibly dysesthesia.

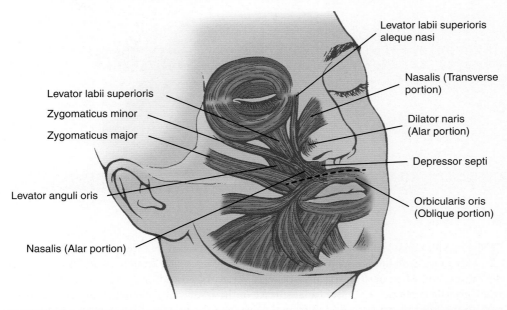

FIGURE 7.1 Facial musculature of importance when performing the maxillary vestibular approach. *Dashed line* is the location of vestibular incision.

Nasolabial Musculature

The attachments of the facial muscles of the nasolabial region may be disrupted during the maxillary vestibular approach. Therefore, these muscles should be properly repositioned during closure to avoid undesirable esthetic changes to the face. The muscles of importance are the nasalis group, the levator labii superioris alaeque nasi, the levator labii superioris, the levator anguli oris, and the orbicularis oris (see Fig. 7.1).

The nasalis group has transverse nasal and alar parts. It originates along the midline of the nasal dorsum and spreads laterally over the external aspect of the upper lateral cartilages where it intermingles with fibers of the levator labii superioris alaeque nasi and the levator labii superioris. Part of the transverse nasalis inserts into the skin at the nasolabial groove, where it intermingles with fibers from the levator labii superioris alaeque nasi and oblique fibers of the orbicularis oris, forming a lateral nasal modiolus. Another portion of the transverse nasalis inserts onto the incisal crest and anterior nasal spine and is in deep contact with the depressor septi muscle. The alar portion is ultimately reflected inward, forming the anterior floor of the nose.

Several muscle groups elevate the upper lip. The levator labii superioris alaeque nasi rises from the frontal process of the maxilla alongside the nose and passes obliquely in two segments. One segment inserts onto the lateral crus of the alar cartilage and skin of the nose, and the other deeper segment extends to the nasal vestibule, blending with fibers of the nasalis muscle, depressor septi, and oblique bands of the orbicularis oris. The levator labii superioris arises from the infraorbital margin of the maxilla beneath the orbicularis oculi. It extends downward and medially, superficial to and intermingling with the orbicularis oris, beneath the skin of the ipsilateral lower philtral columns and the upper lip. The levator anguli oris muscle lies deep to the levator labii superioris and the zygomaticus muscles. It arises from the canine fossa of the maxilla and courses downward and medially to the commissure, where it intermingles with the fibers of the orbicularis oris muscle.

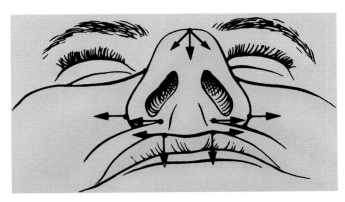

FIGURE 7.2 Effects of the maxillary vestibular approach if simple closure is performed: the nasal tip loses projection, the alar bases widen, and the upper lip rolls inward.

The orbicularis oris muscle consists of three distinct strata. Horizontal fibers extend from one commissure to the other, passing beneath the philtrum. Oblique bands extend from the commissures to the anteroinferior aspect of the nasal septal cartilage, anterior nasal spine, and floor of the nose. The incisal bands extend from the commissures deeply to insert onto the incisive fossa of the maxilla. All these muscles and their investing fascia together contribute significantly to the position and configuration of the lateral nasal and labial regions.

The maxillary vestibular incision and the subperiosteal dissection attendant to this approach cut some of the muscular origins and strip the origins and insertions of most muscles from the bone (Fig. 7.1), causing superolateral retraction of the tissues by the action of the zygomaticus muscles and the natural tendency for muscles to reattach in a shortened position. Lateral displacement of the nasal modiolus causes widening of the alar base with flaring of the alae from unopposed action of the dilator naris. This displacement causes deepening of the alar groove and splaying of the alar bases, nostrils, and nasal tip (see Fig. 7.2). Loss of soft tissue fullness in the nasolabial region results in changes that are similar to those seen in the aging face: thinning and retraction of the upper lip, reduced vermillion exposure, and a more obtuse nasolabial angle. Down-turning of the corner of the mouth may occur when the levators of the upper lip are detached from their origin because the depressors of the mouth will then be unopposed.

Buccal Fat Pad

The buccal fat pad consists of a main body and four extensions: buccal, pterygoid, superficial, and deep temporal. The body is centrally positioned. The buccal extension lies superficially within the cheek, and the pterygoid and temporal extensions are situated more deeply.

The main body of the fat pad is located above the parotid duct and extends along the upper portion of the anterior border of the masseter. It then courses medially to rest on the periosteum of the posterior maxilla (see Fig. 7.3). In this region, the body of the fat pad overlies the uppermost fibers of the buccinator muscle and travels forward along the vestibule overlying the maxillary second molar. Posteriorly, it wraps around the maxilla and travels through the pterygomaxillary fissure, where it is in intimate contact with branches of the internal maxillary artery and the maxillary division of the trigeminal nerve.

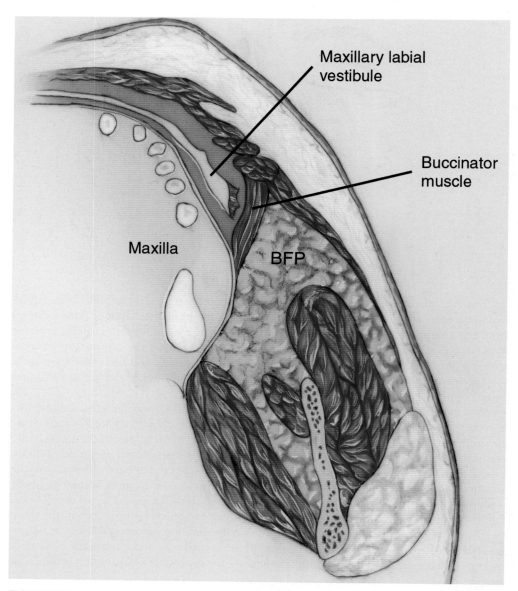

FIGURE 7.3 Axial section through the maxilla at the level of the tooth root apices showing the relation of the buccal fat pad (*BFP*) to the lateral maxilla. Note that the fat pad extends anteriorly to approximately the first molar. Also, posterior to the origin of the buccinator muscle on the maxilla, the buccal fat pad is just lateral to the periosteum.

Maxillary Vestibular Approach

The facial surface of the midface can be exposed using the maxillary vestibular approach. The length of incision and extent of subperiosteal dissection depend on the area of surgical interest and the extent of the surgical intervention. If the area of interest involves only one half of the midface, for instance, with a unilateral zygomaticomaxillary fracture, the incision can be made on one side only, leaving the other side intact (Video 7.1).

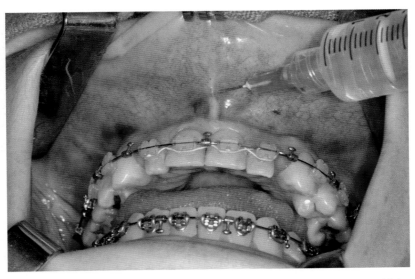

FIGURE 7.4 Photograph showing injection of local anesthesia with a vasoconstrictor into the submucosa.

Technique

➤ STEP 1. Injection of Vasoconstrictor

The oral mucosa, submucosa, and facial muscles are lushly vascularized. Submucosal injection of a vasoconstrictor can dramatically reduce the amount of hemorrhage during incision and dissection (see Fig. 7.4).

➤ STEP 2. Incision

The incision is usually placed approximately 3 to 5 mm superior to the mucogingival junction (see Fig. 7.5). Leaving unattached mucosa on the alveolus facilitates closure. This tissue has many elastic fibers and contracts following incision, although, during closure, the tissue can be grasped and it holds sutures well. The incision should not be made more superior in the anterior region because entrance into the piriform aperture, with puncturing the nasal mucosa, may result. Some individuals have extremely low piriform apertures, which make this possibility a reality. Palpation of the inferior extent of the piriform aperture and/or anterior nasal

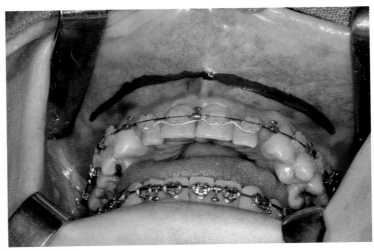

FIGURE 7.5 Photograph showing location of incision, 3 to 5 mm superior to the mucogingival junction.

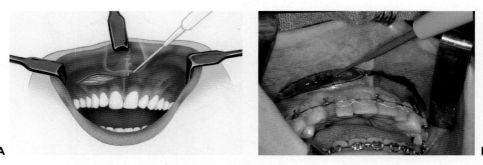

FIGURE 7.6 Illustration **(A)** and photograph **(B)** showing incision through the mucosa, submucosa, facial musculature, and periosteum.

spine ensures incision placement inferior to these structures. In the edentulous maxilla, where atrophy of the alveolar bone brings the alveolar crest and floor of the nose in close apposition, incision along the alveolar crest is an excellent choice.

The incision extends as far posteriorly as necessary to provide exposure, usually up to the first molar tooth, and traverses the mucosa, submucosa, facial muscles, and periosteum (see Fig. 7.6). The mucosa retracts during incision, exposing underlying tissues.

➤ **STEP 3.** Subperiosteal Dissection of Anterior Maxilla and Zygoma

Periosteal elevators are used to elevate the tissues in the subperiosteal plane (see Fig. 7.7). Dissection of the tissues should be carried out in a specific order, first elevating the superior tissues, then the tissues along the piriform aperture, and then the posterior tissues behind the zygomaticomaxillary buttress. While elevating the tissues superiorly in the subperiosteal plane, small perforating vessels are encountered and are easily distinguishable from the infraorbital neurovascular bundle by their size. The infraorbital neurovascular bundle is identified by dissecting medially and laterally to the location of the infraorbital canal, working toward the bundle. After the bundle is located, the periosteum is dissected completely around the foramen. Dissection proceeds superiorly to the infraorbital rim. Subperiosteal dissection along the piriform aperture strips the attachments of the nasolabial musculature, allowing upward and lateral retraction of the muscles.

Subperiosteal dissection proceeds posteriorly to the pterygomaxillary fissure. Perforation of the periosteum at or behind the zygomaticomaxillary buttress produces herniation of the buccal fat pad into the surgical field, which is a nuisance during surgery. A helpful suggestion is to always keep the tip of the periosteal elevator in intimate contact with bone when proceeding

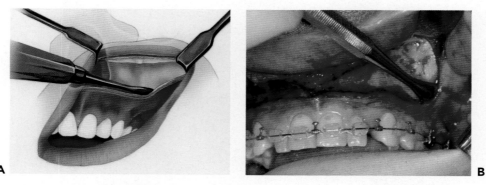

FIGURE 7.7 Illustration **(A)** and photograph **(B)** showing subperiosteal dissection of the maxilla.

posteriorly around the zygomaticomaxillary buttress. The only anatomic hazards are the infra-orbital neurovascular bundle above and posterior superior alveolar vessels along the posterior maxilla, which infrequently cause bleeding.

The entire anterior face of the zygoma can be easily exposed, but reaching the zygomatic arch necessitates detachment of some of the masseter muscle attachments. Sharp dissection is needed to free these tenacious fibers. Dissection below the piriform aperture up the anterior nasal spine should be performed carefully to maintain the integrity of the nasal mucosa. When violated, the nasal mucosa bleeds profusely.

> **STEP 4.** Submucosal Dissection of Nasal Cavity

If it is necessary to strip the nasal mucosa from the lateral wall, floor, or septum of the nose, this maneuver is done carefully, with periosteal or Freer elevators. A forked right-angle retractor is placed over the anterior nasal spine, and superior subperiosteal dissection allows the retractor to retract the septum and nasal mucosa above the level of the anterior nasal spine. A scalpel is used to make a horizontal incision on top of the anterior nasal spine, freeing the cartilaginous septum from the top of the spine and, the attachment of the nasal mucosa from the anterior nasal spine. The rim of the piriform aperture is thin and sharp, and the nasal mucosa is adherent. Periosteal elevators are used to strip the mucosa from the entire circumference of the piriform rim.

Dissection into the nasal cavity is easiest to perform along the lateral wall and floor. The anteroinferior margin of the piriform rim is usually located above the nasal floor. Therefore, after freeing the nasal mucosa from the piriform rim, the elevators should be inserted inferiorly before advancing posteriorly (see Fig. 7.8). Dissection of the lateral wall of the nose is performed by gently inserting a periosteal elevator between the nasal mucosa and the lateral wall of the nasal cavity. It is not advanced deeply until the entire circumference of the lower one half of the piriform has been dissected. The previously taut nasal mucosa can then be relaxed somewhat so that the elevator can be advanced deeper along the lateral wall. The elevator is advanced in a sweeping motion to free the entire lateral wall and floor of its mucosa to the level of the inferior turbinate. The posterior edge of the nasal floor is approximately 45 mm posterior to the piriform aperture and can be felt when the elevator steps off the posterior edge.

Once the lateral wall and floor of the nose are stripped of mucosa, the elevator is placed at the junction of the floor of the nose and the nasal septum. A tenacious attachment of the mucosa to the septal crest of the maxilla must be carefully elevated to prevent perforation. A simple maneuver for stripping the septal mucosa during this approach is to place a Freer elevator along the junction of the septum and the floor of the nose and to twist it so that the edge against the septum is twisted superiorly, freeing the mucosa on the septum.

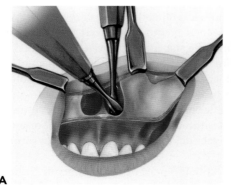
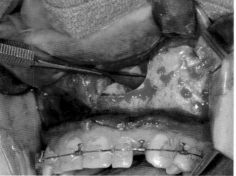

A   **B**

FIGURE 7.8 Illustration **(A)** and photograph **(B)** showing submucosal dissection of the nasal cavity. Note the tip of the periosteal elevator inside the piriform aperture.

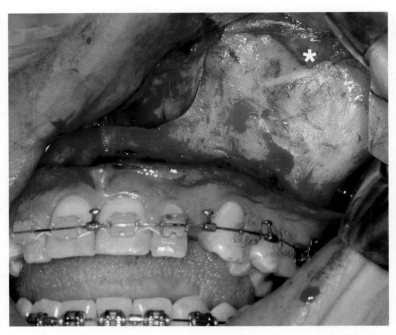

FIGURE 7.9 Photograph showing exposure of entire face of the left anterior maxilla. Note the position of the infraorbital nerve (*).

The entire anterior face of the maxilla is easily exposed using the maxillary vestibular approach (see Fig. 7.9).

➤ **STEP 5.** Closure

Restitution of the nasolabial muscles is performed as three uniform steps during closure of the maxillary vestibular incision. The first step involves identification and resetting of the alar bases, the second involves eversion of the tubercle and vermillion, and the last involves closure of the mucosa.

To help control the width of the alar base, an alar cinch suture is placed prior to suturing the lip. Suture placement is accomplished in one of two ways. In the first, a small-toothed forceps or a single skin hook is placed through the vestibular incision to grasp the insertion of the transverse nasalis muscle. Pulling the instrument medially, allows the change that occurs in the alar base to be seen. A slowly resorbing suture is passed through this tissue, taking care to engage adequate tissue to resist the pull of the suture but not so much tissue that a subcutaneous dimple occurs when the suture is pulled medially. The suture is then passed through the opposite side and temporarily tightened to examine the effect of the medial pull of the alar bases on the nose (see Fig. 7.10). The second method is to evert the tissue into the incision area by pressing the thumb or finger into the alar-facial groove (see Fig. 7.11). A suture can then be passed through the incision, into the tissue, the depth of placement being guided by palpating with the thumb or finger. Whichever method is used to pass the suture through the nasalis muscle, the appearance must be symmetric and the desired curvature and definition of the alar base should be achieved after provisional tying. Tying the suture is delayed until a second suture is passed. The second suture is placed at a higher level or more laterally on the alar base, depending on the desired rotation of the ala. Generally, two sutures are adequate.

A V–Y advancement closure of the maxillary vestibular incision is recommended where the incision was placed across the base of the nose and subperiosteal dissection of the tissues along the piriform aperture was made. While closing the maxillary vestibular incision, a skin hook is used to engage the labial mucosal incision in the midline and pulls it away

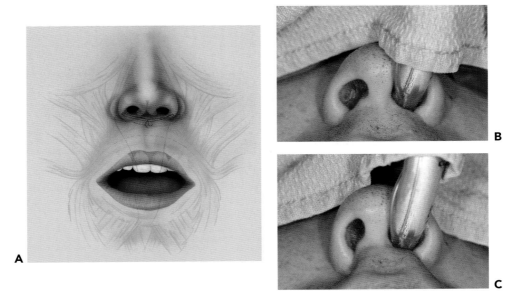

FIGURE 7.10 Illustration **(A)** showing the effect of the alar cinch technique on the width of the alar base. After tying the suture, the alar width is reduced. Photographs before **(B)** and after **(C)** placement of alar cinch suture in a patient. Note the difference after placing the suture.

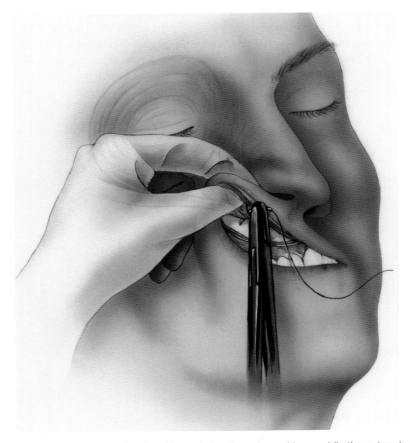

FIGURE 7.11 Tip of the finger (or thumb) everts the lip and nasal base while the suture is passed.

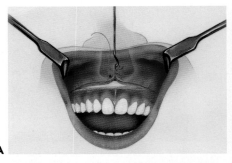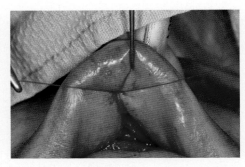

FIGURE 7.12 Illustration **(A)** and photograph **(B)** of V–Y closure of a lip incision. A skin hook is placed in the midline and a slowly resorbing suture is passed through mucosa, submucosa, and muscle on each side and tied. The "Y" portion of the closure is gathered for a length of approximately 1 cm. The lip will be noticeably everted and elevated after placing the suture.

from the maxilla (see Fig. 7.12). Three or four interrupted slowly resorbable sutures are used to gather the lip tissue in the midline. The mucosa, submucosa, and labial musculature are engaged by the needle on either side of the incision and then sutured. In most cases, 1 cm of tissue is closed in this manner, creating a pout in the midline of the lip (see Fig. 7.13). When this step is performed properly, the lip bulges anteriorly in the midline and the exposed vermillion is full. Within 7 to 10 days, this fullness gradually settles and a more normal appearance returns.

After making the vertical limb of the V–Y closure, a single suture is placed across the incision in the midline to assure symmetric closure of the horizontal posterior incisions. When closing the horizontal incision, one should begin in the posterior and work anteriorly with a running resorbable suture (3-0 chromic catgut) through mucosa, submucosa, musculature, and periosteum. The superior aspect of the incision is gradually advanced toward the midline by passing the needle anteriorly in the lower margin of the incision as compared to the upper margin. This maneuver, in addition to the V–Y closure, helps

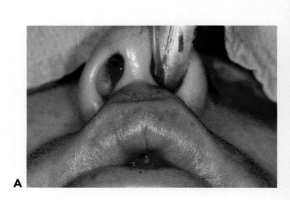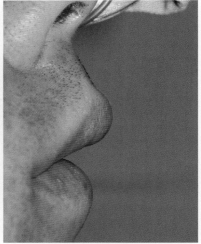

FIGURE 7.13 Frontal **(A)** and lateral **(B)** photographs showing the lip after V–Y closure of the vestibular incision. Notice the "pout" that was created by this technique.

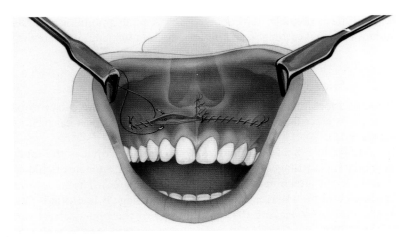

FIGURE 7.14 The remainder of the incision is closed so that the superior edge is pulled anteriorly.

lengthen the relaxed musculature so that it reattaches in its proper position (see Fig. 7.14). From the canine-to-canine area, the suture is passed close to the edges of the incisions to prevent gathering of the mucosa, which will roll the lip inward and reduce the amount of exposed vermillion.

Midfacial Degloving Approach

The degloving approach to the midfacial skeleton can be used to augment the exposure provided by the vestibular approach through the exposure of the external nasal skeleton. The degloving approach combines maxillary vestibular incisions with endonasal incisions. The greatest advantage of the approach is that the scars are hidden (Video 7.2).

Surgical Anatomy

The anatomy of importance to this approach has been described earlier. In addition, knowledge of pertinent nasal anatomy is required. The reader is referred to Chapters 13 and 14 for these details.

Technique

➤ **STEP 1.** Vasoconstriction and Preparation

General anesthesia with oral or submental endotracheal intubation is preferred. It is impossible to perform this approach using nasotracheal intubation.

Infiltration of a vasoconstrictor into the vestibular mucosa is performed as described for the maxillary vestibular approach. In addition, the nose is prepared for surgery. The nasal vibrissae within the vestibules are shaved with a no. 15 scalpel or scissors and the nasal cavity is cleaned with a povidone–iodine solution. A combination of intranasal packs and vasoconstrictor injections help hemostasis during surgery. Nasal packing with a vasoconstrictor (e.g., 4% cocaine, 0.05% oxymetazoline) is placed along the length of the nasal floor, against the turbinates and under the osteocartilaginous roof. Local infiltration of a vasoconstrictor produces hemostasis and assists dissection by separating tissue planes. The infiltration is carried out between the skin of the osteocartilaginous skeleton, trying to deform the overlying skin as little as possible, and submucosally. A small amount is infiltrated between the upper and lower lateral cartilages, and in the membranous septum where the transfixion incision is made.

➤ **STEP 2.** Intranasal Incisions

Three intranasal incisions that are connected to one another are necessary to perform this approach: bilateral intercartilaginous, complete transfixion, and bilateral piriform aperture incisions (see Fig. 7.15).

The *intercartilaginous incision* (limen vestibuli incision) divides the junction of the upper and lower lateral cartilages. The incision traverses the aponeuroticlike fibroareolar tissue that maintains the attachment between them (scroll area). The ala is retracted using a double skin hook and the inferior edge of the alar cartilage is identified. The skin hook elevates the alar cartilages, leaving the inferior edge of the upper lateral cartilage protruding into the vestibule, covered only by the nasal mucosa. An incision is made along the inferior border of the upper lateral cartilage, beginning at the lateral end of the limen vestibuli and extending medially approximately 2 mm caudal to the limen and parallel to it (see Fig. 7.16). It is essential to make the incision 2 to 3 mm caudal to the limen vestibuli to avoid unnecessary scarring at the nasal valve area. The incision is then curved into the membranous septum anterior to the valve area, where it meets the transfixion incision

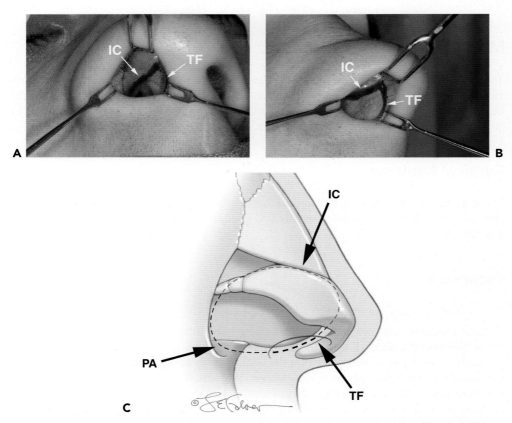

FIGURE 7.15 Intranasal incisions for the facial degloving approach. Frontal photograph **(A)**, lateral photograph **(B)**, and illustration **(C)** showing the three intranasal incisions that are necessary to "free" the nasal tip from the osteocartilaginous skeleton of the nose. *IC*, Intercartilaginous; *TF*, transfixion incision; *PA*, piriform aperture incision.

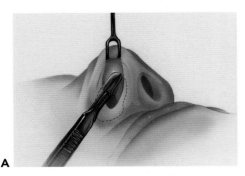
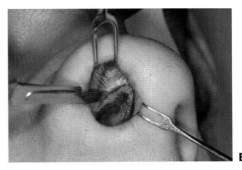
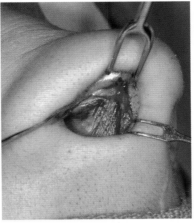

FIGURE 7.16 Intercartilaginous incision. Illustration **(A)** and photograph **(B)** showing an intercartilaginous incision being performed. **C:** Photograph showing the intercartilaginous incision connected to the transfixion incision.

(Fig. 7.16C). The length of the incision must be sufficient so that it extends laterally to the piriform aperture.

A complete *transfixion incision* is made at the caudal end of the septal cartilage and is connected to the intercartilaginous incision. Transfixion is a technique in which the soft tissues overlying the dorsum and columella are separated from the septum. An incision is made along the caudal border of the septal cartilage from the medial end of the intercartilaginous incision toward the anterior nasal spine (see Fig. 7.17). The incision is made all the way to the base of the piriform aperture. Preferably, the incision is placed against the caudal border of the septal cartilage, leaving the membranous septum attached to the columella. Because a complete transfixion incision is necessary, it is made from one side through to the other with the scalpel. It is essential to extend the transfixion incision around the septal angle to permit the release of the alar cartilages from their septal attachments.

The third intranasal incision is along the piriform aperture, connecting the lateral portion of the intercartilaginous incision to the posterior end of the transfixion incision, across the base of the nose at the piriform aperture. Skin hooks are placed along the nasal sill and alae, and a scalpel or a curved beaver blade is used to incise directly to the bone along the rim of the piriform aperture. Alternatively, the incision can be made through the nasal mucosa after the maxillary vestibular incision has been made (see Fig. 7.18). Scissors are

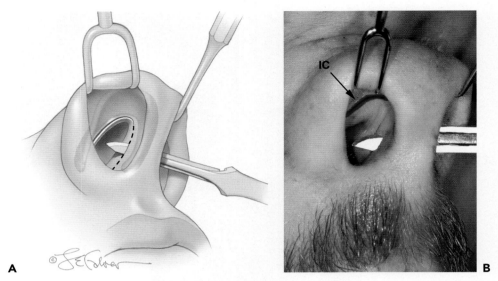

FIGURE 7.17 Transfixion incision. Illustration **(A)** and photograph **(B)** showing incision through the membranous septum along the caudal border of the septum. *IC*, intercartilaginous incision.

inserted and spread to ensure that the internal nasal incisions are now circumvestibular (see Fig. 7.19).

➤ **STEP 3.** Exposure of the Nasal Dorsum and Root

Access to the nasal dorsum and root is gained through the intercartilaginous incision. Once the incision has been made through mucosa, submucosa, aponeurotic tissue, and perichondrium, a sharp subperichondral dissection with a scalpel or a blunt dissection with a sharp scissors frees the soft tissues from the upper lateral cartilages (see Fig. 7.20). The dissection should be within the subperichondral plane to prevent injury to the overlying musculature and blood vessels of the nose. Dissection up to the inferior border of the nasal bones and across the midline to the opposite side is performed through each intercartilaginous incision. Retraction of the freed soft tissues allows a sharp incision to be made with a scalpel through the periosteum at the inferior edge of the nasal bones. Sharp periosteal elevators such as a

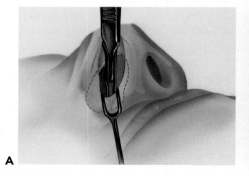
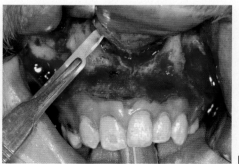

FIGURE 7.18 Piriform aperture incision. **A:** Illustration showing incision from the transfixion incision medially to the intercartilaginous incision laterally along the piriform aperture. **B:** Photograph showing this incision being made from within the maxillary vestibular approach.

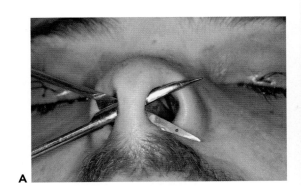

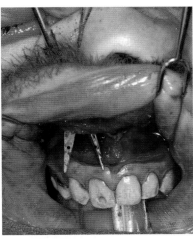

FIGURE 7.19 A: Photograph showing the use of scissors to assure that the transfixion incision is complete and connected to the intercartilaginous incisions. **B:** Photograph showing scissors used to ensure that the piriform rim incision is complete.

Cottle, Joseph, or Freer are useful for subperiosteal dissection of the nasal bones to the level that is necessary for the surgical procedure (Fig. 7.20D). Elevation of the soft tissues laterally to the piriform aperture is also performed so that, when the maxillary vestibular dissection is made, it will easily connect to this pocket.

➤ **STEP 4.** Maxillary Vestibular Incision and Subperiosteal Exposure

The standard incision in the maxillary vestibule as described earlier is made and a sub-periosteal dissection is performed with periosteal elevators to expose the anterior face of the maxilla and zygoma. At the lower portion of the piriform aperture, the entry into the nose in a

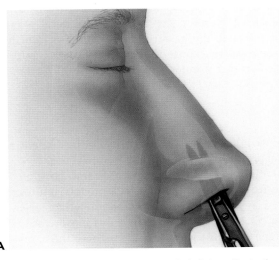

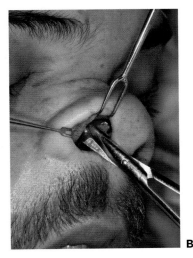

FIGURE 7.20 Exposure of the nasal skeleton. Illustration **(A)** and photographs **(B** and **C)** showing use of scissors inserted through the intercartilaginous incision to dissect the soft tissues from the nasal skeleton. **D:** Illustration showing use of a periosteal elevator to dissect the periosteum from the nasal bones. *(continued)*

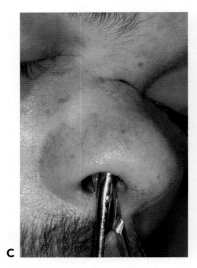
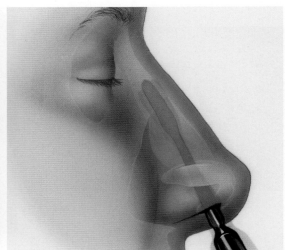

FIGURE 3.20 (*continued*)

subperiosteal manner leads to the circumvestibular incision made in each naris. Subperiosteal dissection along the upper portions of the piriform aperture will connect to the subperiosteal dissection previously performed over the upper lateral cartilages of the nose and nasal bones. Elevation of the lip and columella with a skin hook allows the nasal tip to be "peeled" from the nasal septum and upper lateral cartilages (see Fig. 7.21). Penrose drains can be inserted through the nares into the mouth to use as a retractor of the soft tissues. These can be clipped to the drapes above the forehead to act as self-retaining retractors. The soft tissue mask can be elevated to the level of the nasofrontal suture without difficulty, using periosteal elevators to release any residual connections of soft tissue. Care should be taken not to detach the medial canthal tendons.

➤ STEP 5. Midfacial Osteotomies

Depending upon the needs of the surgical procedure, additional exposure to deeper structures can be attained by midfacial osteotomies. For instance, the nasal pyramid can be removed to provide enhanced access to the nasofrontal duct and/or cribriform plate. The anterior maxilla can be removed to expose the maxillary and/or ethmoid sinuses. Segmental and/or complete Le Fort osteotomies can also be performed from this approach.

➤ STEP 6. Closure

If the medial canthal tendons were removed during the surgery, they must be carefully reattached to their attachments to the frontal process of the maxilla and lacrimal bone.

The soft tissues are then redraped and the nasal tip brought back into position. The intranasal soft tissue incisions can be reapproximated with 4-0 resorbable sutures. The maxillary vestibular incision is closed as described earlier after properly reorienting the nasolabial musculature with an alar cinch suture and possibly a V–Y closure. An external nasal splint is applied to help redrape the soft tissues of the nose onto the nasal skeleton and to help prevent the formation of hematoma (see Chapter 13). Shortened nasal trumpets may be left in the nose for 48 hours to conform the nostrils and to prevent deeper synechiae.

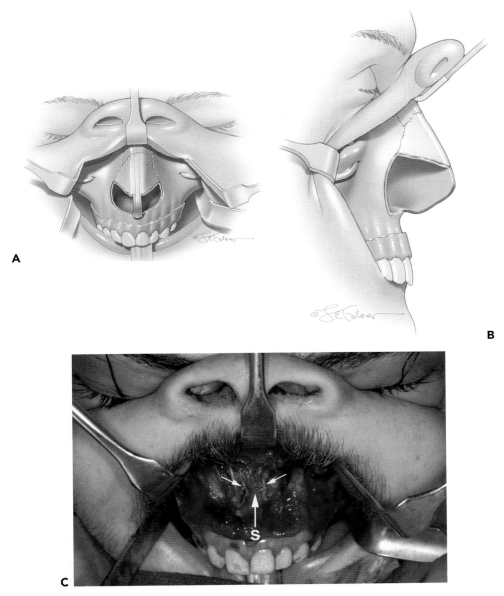

FIGURE 7.21 Exposure of the midface. Frontal **(A)** and lateral **(B)** illustrations of the exposure obtained. **C:** Photograph showing the same. The top retractor is on the nasal bridge and the ones at 10 o'clock and 2 o'clock positions are on the infraorbital rims. *S*, nasal septum; *small arrows* pointing to the septal mucosa where it was severed by the transfixion incision.

Weber-Fergusson Approach to the Midfacial Skeleton

Transoral access to the maxilla and nose might be adequate for a variety of limited neoplastic, inflammatory, or traumatic processes. Greater exposure has historically been obtained through a Weber-Fergusson type incision or a modification of it. The Weber-Fergusson incisions may be used in parts, extended as necessary, incising and dissecting further as the need arises. The external scar from this approach is minimal because it is located between facial esthetic subunits, as long as certain suggestions are followed. These will be noted.

Surgical Anatomy

The surgical anatomy of the lateral cheek area has been described earlier in this chapter; the anatomy of the lip and lateral orbital areas are added here. The orbicularis oris muscle is not a circumferential band in the middle of the upper lip as it is usually portrayed. The fibers of the orbicularis oris insert into the lip in the area of the philtrum. Short and long fibers decussate (see Fig. 7.22A) and add to the bulk of the philtral columns. The levator labii superioris muscles originate *deep to* the orbital portion of the orbicularis oculi muscles and descend *superficial to* the orbicularis oris muscles contributing to the bulk of the lower two-thirds of the philtral columns (Fig. 7.22A and B). Resection of the origin of the levator muscles, as in a high maxillectomy, will always lead to ipsilateral lip drooping which does not occur with inferior excisions of the maxilla. Resuspension of the midface on residual bone will compensate partially for this anatomical deficiency.

The lateral orbital area involves sensory and motor nerve areas. Directly above the prominence of the cheekbone are the exits of the zygomatico-facial and zygomatico-frontal nerves, the end branches for the lacrimal branch of the trigeminal nerve. The infraorbital nerve (Fig. 7.22B) was described earlier and may or may not be transected during the Weber-Fergusson approach, depending upon the needs for exposure and/or requirements of pathologic resection.

Technique

➤ **STEP 1.** Injection of Vasoconstrictor

The injection of local anesthesia with epinephrine and the use of hypotensive general anesthesia techniques reduce the bleeding associated with midfacial surgery. The local anesthesia solution should be injected along the proposed lines of incision once they have been properly marked on the skin. Additional solution can be injected into the pterygomaxillary fissure areas to minimize bleeding from this area.

➤ **STEP 2.** Incision

Each of the Weber-Fergusson incisions will be discussed separately. The dissection may be subperiosteal or supraperiosteal, depending on the procedure and/or tumor behavior.

Lip: The vermillion–cutaneous border should be tattooed with methylene blue before vasoconstrictor injection. A mismatch of even 1 mm is visible at conversational distance. Although incisions have been suggested along the philtral columns with or without small 2 mm steps at the vermillion–cutaneous junction, the most esthetically pleasing incision is

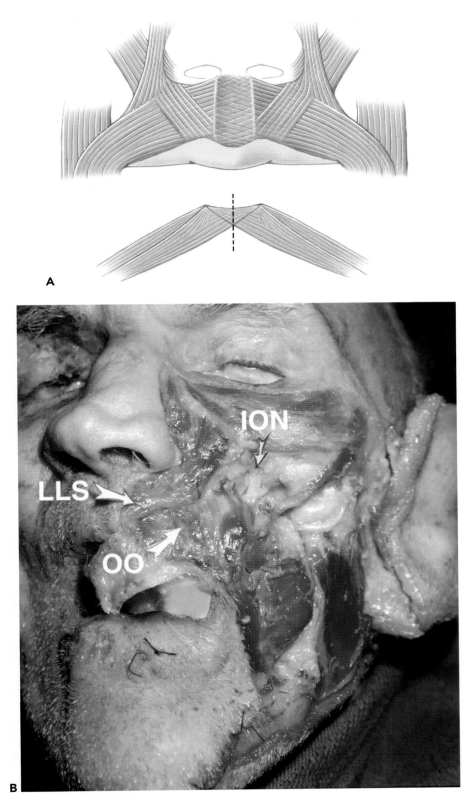

FIGURE 7.22 Anatomy of the upper lip. **A:** Cross-sectional illustration demonstrating how the orbicularis oris muscle fibers insert into the philtral ridges on each side of the lip. The *dashed line* is the location of the incision through the upper lip (see below). **B:** Anatomic dissection showing the levator labii superioris muscle (*LLS*) overlying the orbicularis oris muscle (*OO*). The infraorbital nerve (*ION*) is also shown.

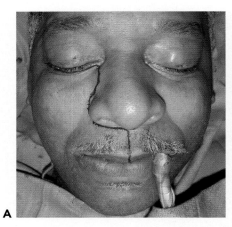
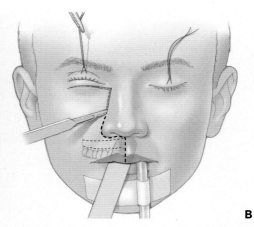

FIGURE 7.23 Photograph **(A)** and illustration **(B)** of the Weber-Fergusson incisions. Note that the incision through the upper lip is made directly in the center of the lip, midway between the philtral columns. **A:** A tongue blade is used to support the lip during incision. The intraoral incisions outlined in *dashed lines* **(B)** can be made either around the cervical margins of the dentition (if present) or in the vestibule depending upon the needs of the procedure.

through the midline (see Fig. 7.23A). The cleanest incision involves a no. 10 blade slicing through the lip onto a flat retractor or tongue blade held beneath the upper lip, giving it support (Fig. 7.23B).

Subnasal: The subnasal extension proceeds around the base of the columella, and just under the roll of the naris. A vertical dart into the naris has been suggested sometimes, but this is superfluous. The incision is made around the alar base, but *not* into it. Keeping the incision 1 to 2 mm lateral to the base will facilitate suturing at closure yet be esthetic.

Lateral nasal: The lateral nasal incision proceeds along the topographic border between the cheek and nose (Fig. 7.23). This topographic border does not follow the resting (relaxed) skin tension lines of the cheek and nose. However, because the topographic border sits in a concavity, incising across it would cause scar tethering. Bleeding from an alar branch of the superior labial artery may occur. The alar and lateral nasal incisions may be used alone for "alotomy" access into the medial nose and ethmoid areas. If more exposure is required, the following additional incision is made.

Extension into the upper eyelid may involve two routes—one in the upper eyelid and one in the lower eyelid.

Upper eyelid extension: If ethmoid exposure is required, extension of the lateral nasal incision superiorly toward the medial eyebrow can be performed. This incision is medial to the medial canthus and the medial canthal tendon can be stripped from its bony origin if necessary. If orbital exenteration is planned along with maxillectomy, the lateral nasal incision is extended into the upper eyelid at the blepharoplasty crease, which ends approximately 6 mm above the lateral canthus. When orbital exenteration is intended, the eyelid skin is elevated superiorly to the superior orbital rim, whose periosteum is incised sharply. From this point, the periosteum may be elevated with a no. 9 periosteal elevator to the orbital apex.

Lower eyelid extension: If access is required only to the maxilla, the lateral nasal incision is extended laterally into the lower eyelid (Fig. 7.23). The level of the incision is decided by the surgeon and can be in a subciliary crease, a subtarsal (mid-eyelid) crease, or the infraorbital rim crease. For most patients, a subtarsal (mid-eyelid) approach is esthetic and resists ectropion when properly supported postoperatively. This extension is easier

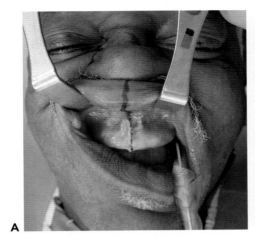
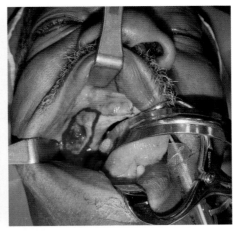

FIGURE 7.24 Photographs showing an edentulous patient whose incisions are placed along the alveolar crest rather than in the vestibule. **A:** The intraoral incision in the midline extends vertically from the lip-splitting incision down to the alveolar crest, where it turns posteriorly. **B:** The soft tissue margins around the pathology are outlined. One incision will be made along the alveolar crest and the other in the vestibule, outlining the pathology. At the conclusion of surgery, advancement of the buccal mucosa to the palatal soft tissues will close the oroantral communication.

to perform from lateral to medial, as described in Chapter 2. The lower eyelid extension may proceed 2.5 cm lateral to the lateral canthus when access to the zygomatic arch is necessary.

Intraoral Incision: The incision along the alveolar process can be made in one of two locations depending upon the requirements of the case: in the vestibular mucosa or around the cervical margins of the teeth (Fig. 7.23B). The maxillary vestibular approach has been discussed earlier in this chapter and can be used in the dentate patient when the alveolar process is to be preserved or when it has to be sacrificed with the overlying gingival soft tissues. However, in many cases where the Weber-Fergusson approach is used, an envelope flap can be employed. For instance, when the alveolar process and portions of the palate are to be removed but the soft tissues are uninvolved in the pathology, the buccal gingival tissues of the envelope flap may be sutured to the remaining palatal soft tissues (if present) at the conclusion of the surgery to prevent an oroantral communication. When preservation of the alveolus is anticipated but there will be a large opening into the maxillary sinus along the anterior maxilla, the incision should be placed around the cervical margins of the teeth (envelope flap) so that closure of the soft tissue is over sound hard tissues rather than over an osseous defect.

When there are large edentulous spaces, the vestibular incision should be *moved inferiorly to the crest of the alveolar ridge*. This maneuver will compensate for alveolar resorption, eliminate most potential oroantral fistulas, and improve denture retention by eliminating a scar band in the vestibule (see Fig. 7.24).

➤ **STEP 3.** Dissection of Flap From Maxilla

Once the skin had been incised, the flap is elevated from the face of the maxilla either supra-or subperiosteally, depending upon the requirements of the procedure and/or requirements of the pathology (see Fig. 7.25). If a subperiosteal dissection is possible, periosteal elevators are used to strip this tissue from the bone. If a supraperiosteal dissection is required, the flap can be dissected from the periosteum with a scalpel, using skin hooks to maintain outward traction on the flap.

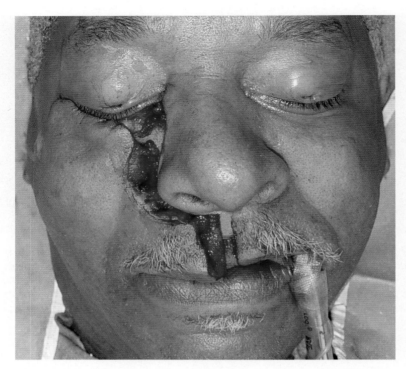

FIGURE 7.25 Photograph after completion of incisions and initial dissection of the flap.

When the infraorbital neurovascular bundle is encountered during flap elevation, it can be preserved or transected depending upon the surgical requirements. If the bundle is to be preserved, the bundle is freed from the surrounding periosteum using sharp pointed scissors. The neurovascular bundle can be dissected into the flap for 1 to 2 cm if necessary to facilitate mobilization of the flap (see Fig. 7.26).

If the infraorbital nerve is to be sacrificed, it is incised at the foramen. This provides great mobility of the facial flap well onto the body of the zygoma (see Fig. 7.27).

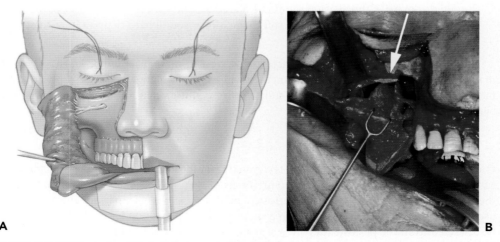

FIGURE 7.26 Illustration **(A)** and photograph **(B)** of infraorbital nerve preservation (*arrow*). The resection osteotomy margin was just inferior to it. The nerve was dissected into the soft tissues of the cheek, providing mobility of the flap.

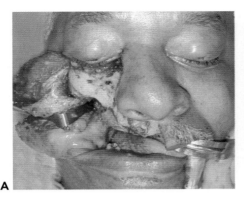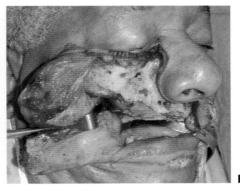

FIGURE 7.27 Frontal **(A)** and lateral **(B)** photographs showing exposed anterior maxilla after dissection of the buccal flap from the anterior maxilla. The dissection in this case was subperiosteal except over the lesion (in alveolus), where it was supraperiosteal. The infraorbital nerve has been sacrificed in this case.

➤ **STEP 4.** Closure

Depending upon the surgical requirements, the raw soft tissue margin on the inside of the cheek flap can be grafted with split-thickness skin (see Fig. 7.28). This is especially helpful if a supraperiosteal dissection along the anterior maxilla was performed and/or if there is a large oroantral communication after surgery, for instance, after a hemimaxillectomy.

Closure of large facial dissections demands restoration of fixed points to prevent distortion from loss of skeletal support due to tumor resection, as well as from dissection of the

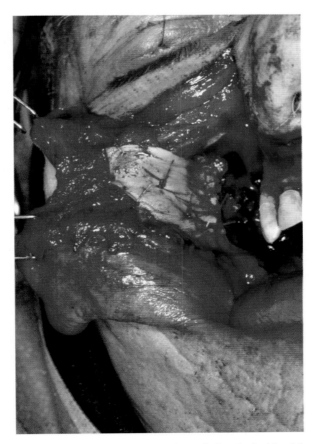

FIGURE 7.28 Photograph of split-thickness skin graft applied to the inside of the cheek flap.

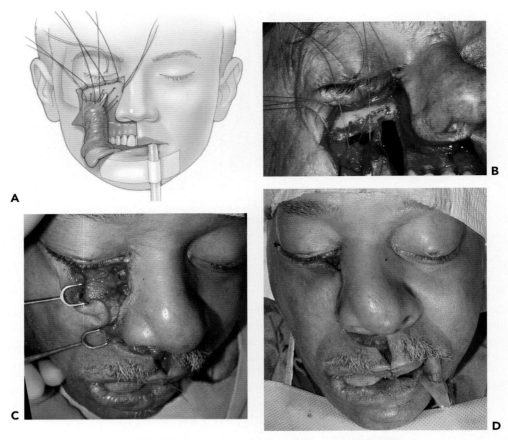

FIGURE 7.29 Resuspension of cheek flap to bony landmarks. Illustration **(A)** and photograph **(B)** showing the suture resuspension of the cheek flap to the infraorbital rim and piriform margin by holes drilled through them. **C:** Photograph after tightening the suspension sutures. Note that the deep tissues have been secured back into their proper positions. **D:** Photograph showing that there is no tension on the skin after appropriate resuspension.

flap from its bony origins. Transnasal suturing (alar cinch is described in the preceding text for vestibular approach) should be performed when the entire piriform region is released. Large flaps should also be pexed to deeper fixed structures. The medial flap should be pexed with slowly resorbing or nonresorbing sutures to the piriform rim by drilling holes through the bony rim to accept the sutures (see Fig. 7.29). The superomedial edge to the flap should be pexed to the medial orbital/nasal rims in a similar manner, or through the canthal tendon and/or periosteum if there is no remaining bone. Holes are drilled through the infraorbital rim to suspend the lateral cheek tissues. Failure to properly suspend the flap to the remaining stable skeletal anatomy leads to ectropion, widening of the scar and/ or midfacial drooping.

A suture is then passed through the mucocutaneous junction of the upper lip to properly realign this important landmark (Fig. 7.29D). The intraoral closure, if planned, is then performed. If the alveolar process has been removed, it is often possible to advance and suture the buccal mucosa to the palatal mucosa and to close an oroantral communication (see Fig. 7.30).

The skin and upper lip are then closed in layers (see Fig. 7.31).

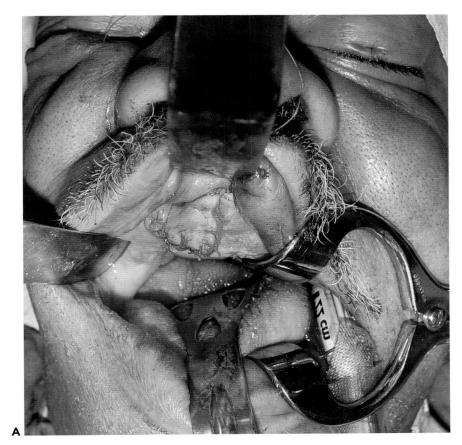

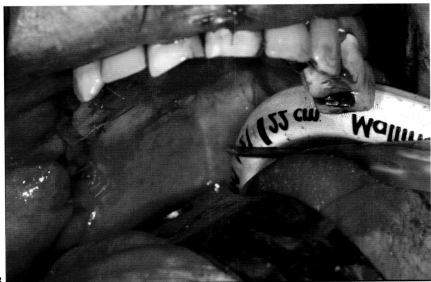

FIGURE 7.30 Intraoral closure. Two examples where the buccal mucosa has been undermined, advanced, and sutured to the palatal mucosa **(A** and **B)**.

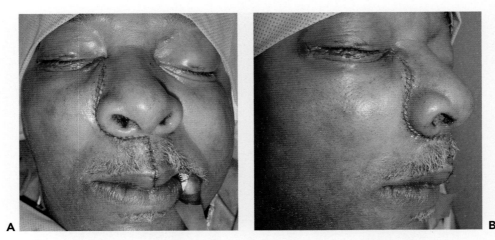

FIGURE 7.31 Skin closure. Frontal **(A)** and lateral **(B)** photographs showing closure of the skin and upper lip.

8

Mandibular Vestibular Approach

The mandibular vestibular approach is useful in a wide variety of procedures. It allows relatively safe access to the entire facial surface of the mandibular skeleton, from the condyle to the symphysis. One advantage of this approach is the ability to constantly assess the dental occlusion during surgery. The greatest benefit to the patient is the hidden intraoral scar. The approach is also relatively rapid and simple, although access is limited in some regions, such as the lower border of the mandible at the angle and parts of the ramus. Complications are few but include mental nerve damage and lip malposition, both of which are minimized with the use of proper technique.

Surgical Anatomy

Mental Nerve

The only neurovascular structure of any significance that must be negotiated during procedures in the mandibular body/symphysis region is the mental neurovascular bundle. The artery and vein that accompany the mental nerve are insignificant from a surgical standpoint. The mental nerve is a terminal branch of the inferior alveolar nerve (mandibular nerve), and is sensory to the skin and mucosa of the lower lip, the skin in the region of the chin, and the facial gingiva of the anterior teeth.

The mental nerve exits the mental foramen that is located midway between the alveolar and basal borders of the mandible and is usually below or slightly anterior to the second bicuspid tooth (see Fig. 8.1). The mental nerve divides under the depressor anguli oris muscle into three main branches; one descends to the skin of the chin and the other two ascend to the skin and mucous membrane of the lower lip and gingiva. The branching pattern is variable however, and several finer branches may be noted. As the branches enter the lower lip, they become superficial and can usually be seen just beneath the mucosa of the lower lip when it is everted.

Facial Vessels

The facial artery and vein are usually not encountered during the mandibular vestibular approach unless dissection through the periosteum occurs in the region of the mandibular antegonial notch.

The facial artery arises from the external carotid artery in the carotid triangle of the neck. At or close to its origin, it is crossed by the posterior belly of the digastric muscle, the stylohyoid muscles, and the hypoglossal nerve. In the submandibular triangle, the facial artery ascends deep to the submandibular gland, grooving its deep and superior aspect, and then passes superficially to reach the inferior border of the mandible. As the

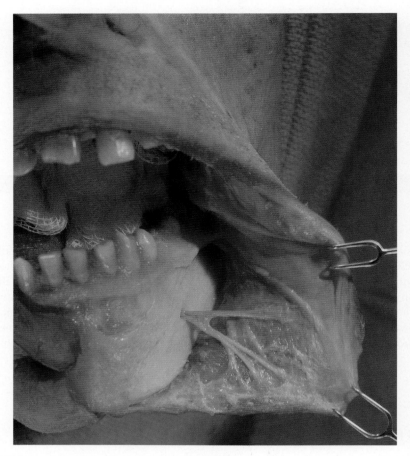

FIGURE 8.1 Anatomic dissection of mental nerve branches.

artery crosses the mandible at the anterior border of the masseter muscle, it is covered on its superficial surface by skin and platysma muscle, and its pulsations can be felt at this location.

The facial vein is the drainage of the angular and ultimately labial vessels. It is usually located more posterior and superficial to the artery. Of surgical significance, however, is the fact that the facial artery and vein are close to the mandible in the region of the inferior border. The only structure that separates the vessels from the bone is the periosteum (see Fig. 8.2).

Mentalis Muscle

The only muscle of facial expression that is important from a surgical standpoint when using the mandibular vestibular approach is the mentalis muscle. All the other muscles of facial expression are stripped from the mandible by subperiosteal dissection and are readily reattached with soft tissue closure. The mentalis muscle is unique however, in that it is the only elevator of the lower lip and chin. If this muscle is not properly repositioned during closure, the chin will "droop" and the lower lip will take on a lifeless, sagging appearance, exposing more lower teeth.

The mentalis muscles are paired, small, conical muscles arising from the mandible, beginning at the midroot level of the lower incisor teeth and continuing inferiorly to a point below the apices. The muscles are separated from one another by a firm septum and adipose tissue (see Fig. 8.3).

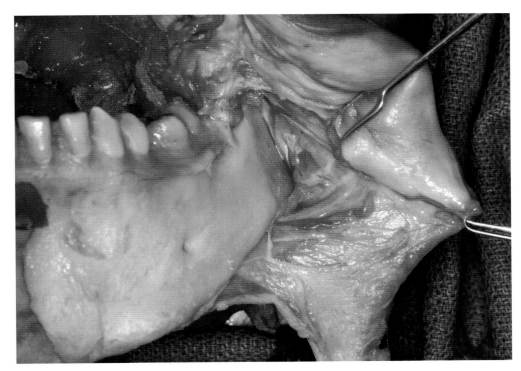

FIGURE 8.2 Anatomic dissection of the mandibular body showing relation of facial vessels to bone. The only tissue between them is the periosteum.

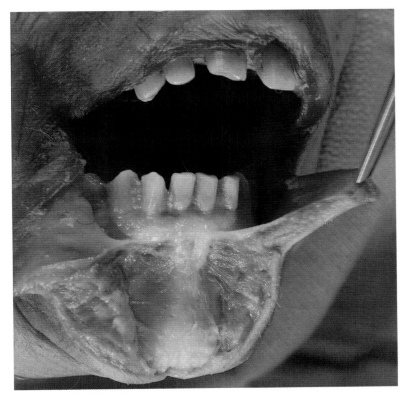

FIGURE 8.3 Anatomic dissection showing cross section of soft tissues of the chin. Note the direction of the mentalis muscle fibers.

At the inferior portion of its origin, the mentalis muscle attaches lateral to the mental trigone. The fibers of this muscle pass from their origin inferiorly, inserting into the skin of the chin at the soft tissue chin prominence. The most superior fibers are the shortest and pass almost horizontally into the skin of the upper chin. The lower fibers are the longest and pass obliquely or vertically to the skin at the lower part of the chin. The origin of the mentalis muscle determines the depth of the labial sulcus in the anterior portion of the mouth. The mentalis muscle is innervated by the marginal mandibular branch of the facial nerve.

Buccal Fat Pad

The buccal fat pad consists of a main body and four extensions: buccal, pterygoid, pterygomandibular, and temporal. The body is centrally positioned. The buccal extension lies superficially within the cheek, while the pterygoid, pterygomandibular, and temporal extensions are more deeply situated.

The buccal extension is the most superficial segment of the fat pad and imparts fullness to the cheek. It enters the cheek below the parotid duct and extends along the anterior border of the masseter as it descends into the mandibular retromolar region. It overlies the main portion of the buccinator muscle as it crosses the cheek. In the cheek, the fat pad is anterior to the ramus. Its caudal extension intraorally is on a plane tangential with the occlusal surface of the mandibular third molar (see Fig. 8.4). Its anterior limit is marked by the facial vessels, which are in the same plane as the buccal fat pad. The parotid duct lies superficial to the fat pad and then penetrates the fat pad and buccinator to enter the oral cavity opposite the second molar.

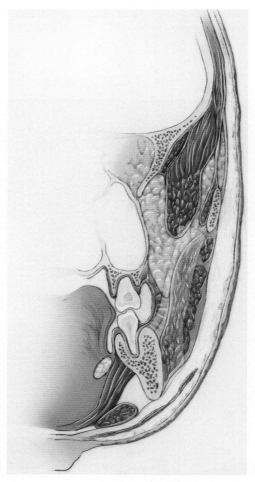

FIGURE 8.4 Relation between the buccal fat pad and the retromolar region. Note that the fat extends inferiorly to just above the occlusal plane. Incisions made through the buccinator muscle superior to the occlusal plane will cause entry into the fat pad.

The buccal extension of the fat pad is limited by the masseteric fascia. A deep extension of the masseteric fascia blends with the fascia along the lateral surface of the buccinator. This fascial layer lines the deep surface of the buccal fat that is in contact with the buccinator.

Technique

For demonstration purposes, the technique subsequently described is that used to expose the entire facial surface of the mandible. The length of the incision and the extent of subperiosteal dissection, however, depend on the area of interest and the extent of surgical intervention (Video 8.1). *While the vestibular approach is used for patients who have teeth, when large segments of teeth are absent the surgeon should consider incisions along the alveolar crest as opposed to vestibular ones.*

➤ **STEP 1.** Injection of Vasoconstrictor

The oral mucosa, submucosa, and facial muscles are lushly vascularized. Submucosal injection of a vasoconstrictor can remarkably reduce the amount of hemorrhage during incision and dissection.

➤ **STEP 2.** Incision

In the anterior region, from canine to canine, the lower lip is everted and a scalpel or electrocautery is used to incise mucosa. The incision is curvilinear, extending anteriorly out into the lip, leaving 10 to 15 mm of mucosa attached to the gingiva (see Fig. 8.5). It is important

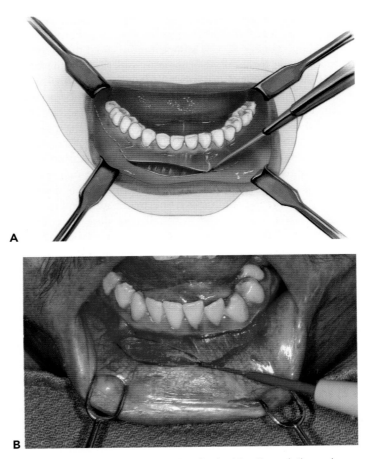

FIGURE 8.5 A: Illustration and **(B)**, photograph showing incision through the oral mucosa in the anterior region out in the lip, exposing the underlying mentalis muscle fibers.

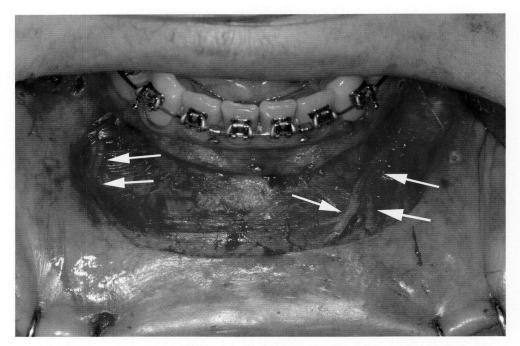

FIGURE 8.6 Photograph showing branches of the mental nerves (*arrows*) just deep to the mucosa.

to incise only through the mucosa because mental nerve branches that extend into the upper lip are often seen just below the mucosa (see Fig. 8.6). Once through the mucosa, the underlying mentalis muscles are clearly visible. The muscle fibers are sharply incised in an oblique approach to the mandible (see Fig. 8.7). It is important to avoid the mental nerve during the incision. The incision should therefore be made more superiorly in the canine and premolar region (see Fig. 8.8). Any incision placed more inferior in the canine/premolar region may sever branches of the mental nerve. The scalpel should therefore be oriented perpendicular to the bone when incising above the mental foramen to prevent incision of this nerve. When bone is encountered, there should be an ample amount of mentalis muscle remaining on its origin for holding deep sutures at closure (see Fig. 8.9).

In the body and posterior portion of the mandible, the incision is placed 3 to 5 mm inferior to the mucogingival junction (see Fig. 8.10). Leaving unattached mucosa on the alveolus facilitates closure. The posterior extent of the incision is made over the external oblique ridge, traversing mucosa, submucosa, buccinator muscle, buccopharyngeal fascia, and periosteum (Fig. 8.5A). The incision is usually no more superior than the occlusal plane of the mandibular teeth to help prevent herniation of the buccal fat pad into the surgical field, a nuisance during surgery. The buccal portion of the buccal fat pad is usually not more inferior than the level of the occlusal plane (Fig. 8.4). Placement of the incision at this level also may spare the buccal artery and nerve, although their damage is more a nuisance than a clinical problem. If the buccal artery is severed, bleeding is easily controlled by coagulation.

In the edentulous mandible, the incision is made along the alveolar crest, splitting the attached gingiva. Placement in this location facilitates closure and minimizes risk to the mental nerve. Alveolar atrophy brings the inferior alveolar neurovascular bundle and the mental foramen to the superior surface of the bone. In these instances, crestal incisions behind and in front of the mental foramen, which is easily located by palpation, are joined following subperiosteal dissection to identify the exact location of the mental nerve. Posteriorly, the incision leaves the crest at the second molar region and extends laterally to avoid the lingual nerve, which may be directly over the third molar area. Placing the incision over the ascending ramus helps to avoid the lingual nerve.

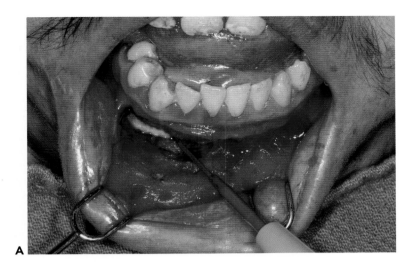

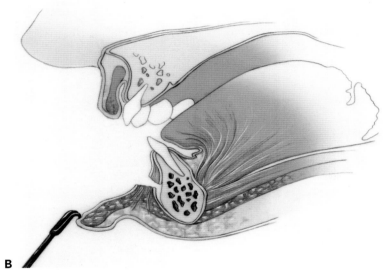

FIGURE 8.7 Photograph showing incision of the mentalis muscle in an oblique direction until bone is encountered **(A)**. **B:** Cross section of the symphysis showing the path of dissection.

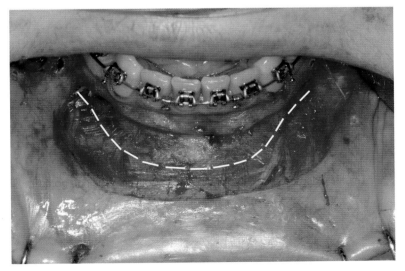

FIGURE 8.8 Photograph demonstrating the line of incision (*dashed line*) through the mentalis muscles. Note that the posterior extent of the incision is in a higher location on the mandible to avoid the mental nerves, which are easily seen in this photograph.

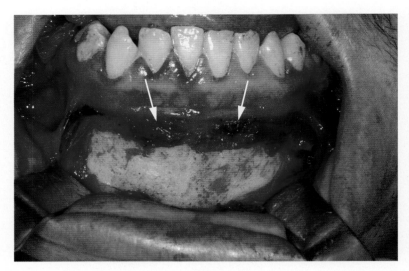

FIGURE 8.9 Photograph showing the severed origin of the mentalis muscles still attached to the mandible.

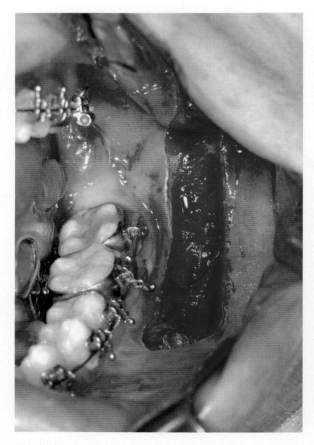

FIGURE 8.10 Photograph showing incision location when vestibular approach is used to expose the ramus and posterior body of the mandible. Note that there is some unattached mucosa remaining along the attached gingiva to facilitate closure.

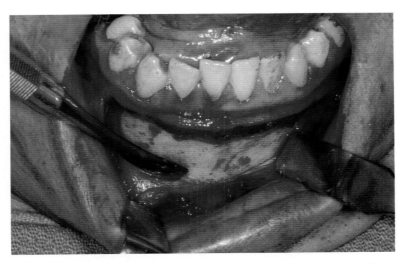

FIGURE 8.11 Photograph showing use of a periosteal elevator to strip the mentalis muscle in the subperiosteal plane from the anterior mandible.

➤ **STEP 3.** Subperiosteal Dissection of the Mandible

The mentalis muscle is stripped from the mandible in a subperiosteal plane (see Fig. 8.11). Retraction of the labial tissues is facilitated by stripping them off the inferior border of the symphysis. Subperiosteal dissection of the mandibular body is relatively simple compared to that of the symphysis because there are fewer Sharpey fibers inserting into the bone. Controlled dissection and reflection of the mental neurovascular bundle facilitates retraction of the soft tissues away from the mandible. The periosteum is totally freed circumferentially around the mental foramen. Retracting the facial tissues laterally will gently tense the mental nerve. Using a scalpel, the surgeon then incises the stretched periosteum longitudinally, paralleling the nerve fibers (see Fig. 8.12A and B) in two or three locations. The sharp end of a periosteal elevator teases the periosteum away from the mental foramen. Any remaining periosteal attachments are dissected free with sharp scissors (Fig. 8.12C and D). This stripping allows mobilization of the branches of the mental nerve, facilitating facial retraction and augmenting exposure of the mandible (Fig. 8.12E and F). Dissection can then proceed posteriorly along the lateral surface of the mandibular body/ramus. The surgeon should stay within the periosteal envelope to prevent lacerating the facial vessels, which are just superficial to the periosteum (Fig. 8.2).

Subperiosteal dissection along the anterior edge of the ascending ramus strips the buccinator attachments, allowing the muscle to retract upward, minimizing the chance of herniation of the buccal fat pad (Fig. 8.4). Temporalis muscle fibers may be stripped easily by inserting the sharp end of a periosteal elevator between the fibers and the bone as high on the coronoid process as possible, and stripping downward (see Fig. 8.13). A notched right-angle retractor (see Fig. 8.14) may be placed on the anterior border of the coronoid process to retract the mucosa, buccinator, and temporalis tendon superiorly during stripping. Stripping some of the tissue from the medial side of the ramus will widen the access. After stripping the upper one third of the coronoid process, a curved Kocher clamp can be used as a self-retaining retractor grasping the coronoid process.

While the buccal tissues are retracted laterally with a right-angle retractor, the masseter muscle is stripped from the lateral surface of the ramus (Fig. 8.13). Sweeping the periosteal elevator superoinferiorly strips the muscle cleanly from the bone. Although direct visualization may be poor, the posterior and inferior borders of the mandible are readily stripped of pterygomasseteric fibers using periosteal elevators, J-strippers, or both. Dissection can continue superiorly, exposing the condylar neck and the entire sigmoid notch. To maintain exposure

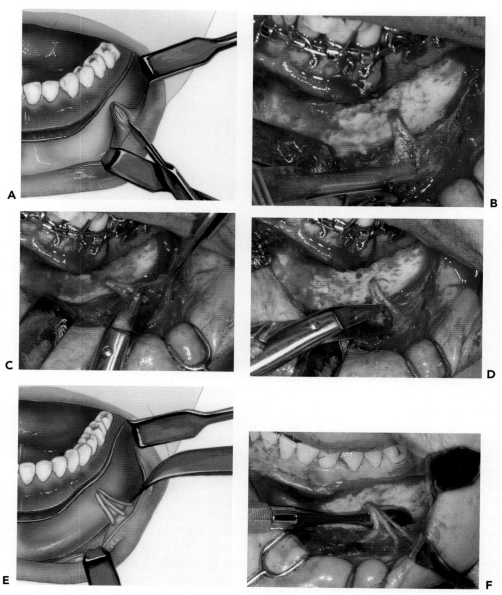

FIGURE 8.12 Dissection of the mental nerves. **A:** Illustration and **(B)** photograph showing incision of the periosteum that covers the nerve branches. **C:** Photograph showing dissection of the periosteum from the nerve branches. **D:** Photograph showing dissection of individual branches of the mental nerve with scissors to facilitate mobilization. **E:** Illustration showing the branches of the mental nerve dissected from their enveloping periosteum. **F:** Photograph showing use of a periosteal elevator to strip the periosteum below the mental foramen. Note that the branches of the mental nerve have been freed and are quite mobile.

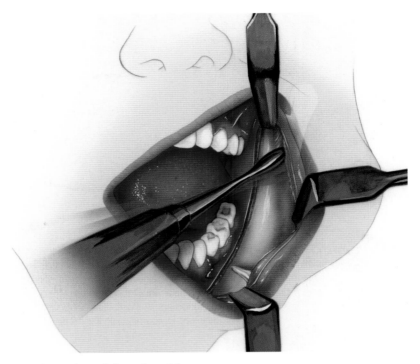

FIGURE 8.13 Subperiosteal dissection of the ramus.

of the ramus, Bauer retractors (see Fig. 8.15) inserted into the sigmoid notch and/or under the inferior border are useful (see Fig. 8.16). The LaVasseur-Merrill retractor is another useful device that slides behind and clutches the posterior border of the mandible to hold the masseter in a lateral position.

➤ **STEP 4.** Closure

Closure is adequate in one layer, except in the anterior region. Closure is begun in the posterior areas with resorbable suture. The pass of the needle should grab mucosa, submucosa, the cut edge of the facial muscles, and the periosteum, if possible. A simple mucosal closure is inadequate because it allows retraction of the facial muscles, which will heal in an abnormally

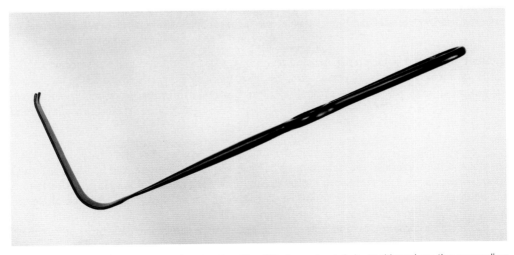

FIGURE 8.14 Notched right-angle retractor. The "V"-shaped notch is positioned on the ascending ramus and the retractor is pulled superiorly to retract tissues.

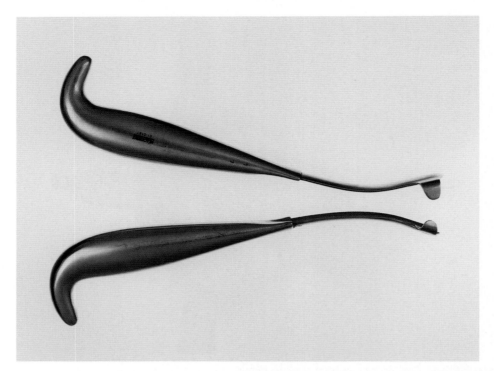

FIGURE 8.15 Bauer retractors. The flanges at right angle to the shaft are used to engage the sigmoid notch and/or inferior border of the mandible, allowing retraction of the masseter muscle.

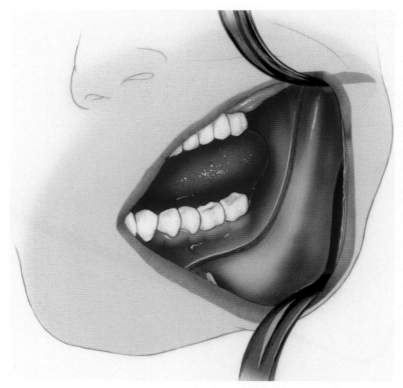

FIGURE 8.16 Exposure after insertion of Bauer retractors. Note the flange of one retractor is in the sigmoid notch and the flange of the other is under the inferior border of the mandible.

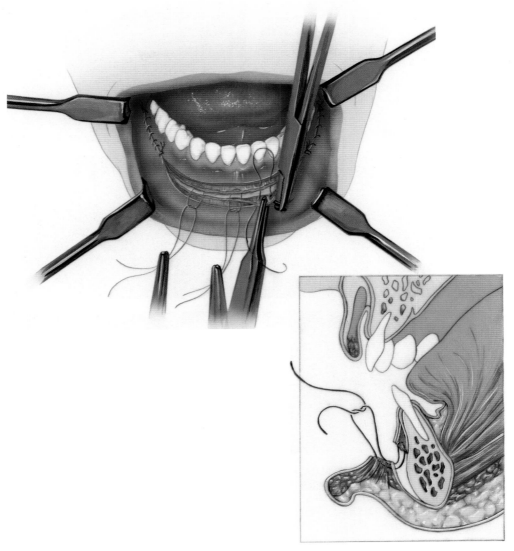

FIGURE 8.17 Closure of the posterior incision is performed in one layer. In the anterior region, delayed sutures are placed in the mentalis muscle prior to mucosal closure.

low position along the mandible. Closure is continued anteriorly to the area of the cuspid tooth. At this point, the suture is tied (see Fig. 8.17). It is imperative that the mentalis muscle is firmly reattached to its origin to prevent ptosis of the lip and chin. A minimum of three deep resorbable sutures are placed in the mentalis muscle to reapproximate the cut edges (Fig. 8.17). To facilitate suturing the mentalis muscle, the lip is everted to expose the incised insertion of the muscle (see Fig. 8.18A). The incised origin of the mentalis muscle is also identified (Fig. 8.18A). A slowly resorbing suture is then placed through the insertion and the origin of each mentalis muscle in a delayed manner (Fig. 8.18B and C), followed by another suture in the midline (Fig. 8.18D). Pressure should be applied in the labiomental crease to provide support while tying of the sutures. Once tied, the lip should be tightly adapted to the mandible (Fig. 8.18E). The mucosa is then closed with a running resorbable suture.

A suspension dressing, such as elastic tape, is useful for several days after the mandibular buccal vestibular approach has been performed, to prevent hematoma and to maintain the position of the repositioned facial muscles (Fig. 8.18F).

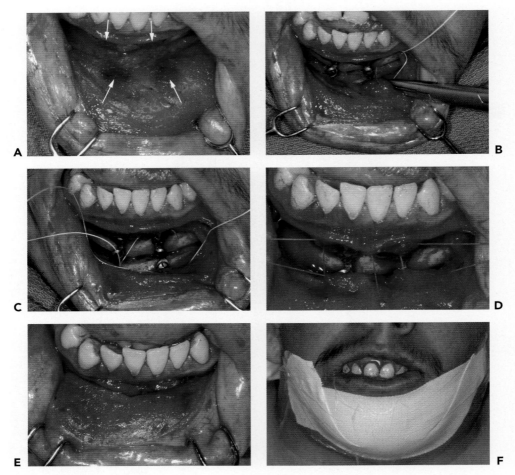

FIGURE 8.18 Photographs showing a demonstration of closure of the vestibular approach to the anterior mandible. **A:** Identification of the incised origin (*upper arrows*) and insertion (*lower arrows*) of the mentalis muscle. **B:** Slowly resorbing suture is passed through the incised insertion of the mentalis muscle. **C:** The suture is then passed through the incised origin. **D:** Three delayed sutures have been placed, one in each muscle and one in the midline. **E:** Appearance after tying the sutures. **F:** Elastic support dressing is placed at the conclusion of surgery.

SECTION 5

Transfacial Approaches to the Mandible

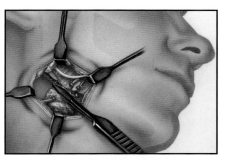
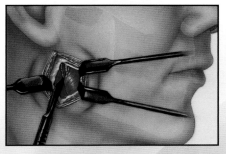
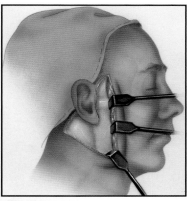

The mandible can be exposed by surgical approaches using incisions placed on the skin of the face. The position of the incisions and anatomy vary depending on the region of the mandible that is approached. Because there are almost no anatomic hazards in the transfacial exposure of the mandibular symphysis, this approach is not presented. The focus of this section is on the submandibular, retromandibular, and rhytidectomy approaches. All these are used to expose the posterior regions of the mandible and all must negotiate important anatomic structures. Approaches to the temporomandibular joint are presented in Section 6.

9

Submandibular Approach

The submandibular approach is one of the most useful approaches to the mandibular ramus and posterior body region, and is occasionally referred to as the *Risdon approach*. This approach may be used for obtaining access to a myriad of mandibular osteotomies, angle/body fractures, and even condylar fractures and temporomandibular joint (TMJ) ankylosis. Descriptions of the approach differ on some points, but in all the incision is made below the inferior border of the mandible (Video 9.1).

Surgical Anatomy

Marginal Mandibular Branch of the Facial Nerve

After the facial nerve divides into temporofacial and cervicofacial branches, the marginal mandibular branch originates and extends anteriorly and inferiorly within the substance of the parotid gland. The marginal mandibular branch or branches, which supply motor fibers to the facial muscles in the lower lip and chin, represent the most important anatomic hazard while performing the submandibular approach to the mandible. Studies have shown that the nerve passes below the inferior border of the mandible only in very few individuals (see Fig. 9.1). In the Dingman and Grabb classic dissection of 100 facial halves, the marginal mandibular branch was almost 1 cm below the inferior border in 19% of the specimens (1). Anterior to the point where the nerve crossed the facial artery, all dissections in the above study displayed the nerve above the inferior border of the mandible.

Ziarah and Atkinson (2) found more individuals in whom the marginal mandibular branch passed below the inferior border. In 53% of 76 facial halves, they found the marginal mandibular branch passing below the inferior border before reaching the facial vessels, and in 6%, the nerve continued for a further distance of almost 1.5 cm before turning upward and crossing the mandible. The farthest distance between a marginal mandibular branch and the inferior border of the mandible was 1.2 cm. In view of these findings, most surgeons recommend that the incision and deeper dissection be at least 1.5 cm below the inferior border of the mandible.

Another important finding of the study by Dingman and Grabb (1) was that only 21% of the individuals had a single marginal mandibular branch between the angle of the mandible and the facial vessels (see Fig. 9.2); 67% had two branches (Fig. 9.1), 9% had three branches, and 3% had four.

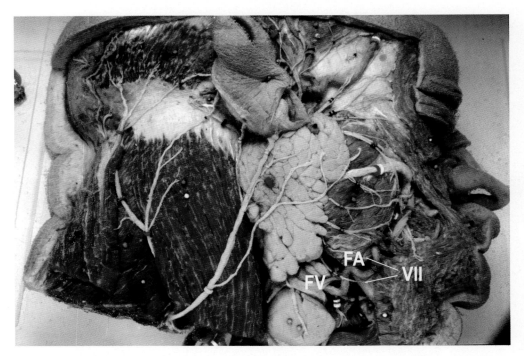

FIGURE 9.1 Anatomic dissection of the lateral face showing the relation of the parotid gland, submandibular gland, facial artery (*FA*) and vein (*FV*), and marginal mandibular branches of the facial nerve (*VII*). Two marginal mandibular branches are present in this specimen, one below the inferior border of the mandible.

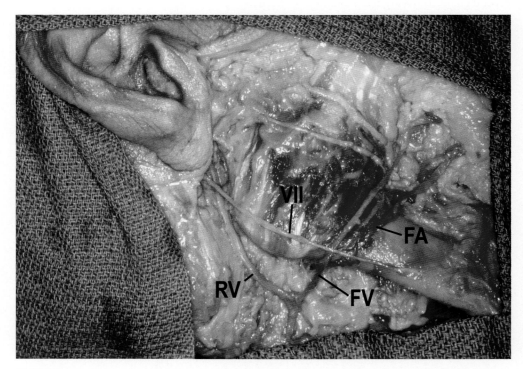

FIGURE 9.2 Anatomic dissection of the lateral face showing the relation of the submandibular gland, facial artery (*FA*) and vein (*FV*), retromandibular vein (*RV*), and marginal mandibular branch of the facial nerve (*VII*) (parotid gland has been removed). Only one marginal mandibular branch is present in this specimen and it is superior to the inferior border of the mandible.

Facial Artery

After it originates from the external carotid artery, the facial artery follows a cervical course during which it is carried upward medial to the mandible and in fairly close contact with the pharynx. It runs superiorly, deep to the posterior belly of the digastric and stylohyoid muscles, and then crosses above them to descend on the medial surface of the mandible, grooving or passing through the submandibular salivary gland as it rounds the lower border of the mandible. It is visible on the external surface of the mandible around the anterior border of the masseter muscle (Figs. 9.1 and 9.2). Above the inferior border of the mandible, it lies anterior to the facial vein and is tortuous.

Facial Vein

The facial (anterior facial) vein is the primary venous outlet of the face. It begins as the angular vein, in the angle between the nose and eye. It generally courses along with the facial artery above the level of the inferior mandibular border, but it is posterior to the artery (Figs. 9.1 and 9.2). Unlike the facial artery, the facial vein runs across the surface of the submandibular gland to end in the internal jugular vein.

Technique

➤ **STEP 1.** Preparation and Draping

Pertinent landmarks on the face, useful during dissection, should be left exposed throughout the procedure. For surgeries involving the mandibular ramus/angle, the corner of the mouth and lower lip should be exposed within the surgical field anteriorly and the ear, or at least the ear lobe, posteriorly. These landmarks help the surgeon to mentally visualize the course of the facial nerve and to see whether the lip moves if stimulated.

➤ **STEP 2.** Marking the Incision and Vasoconstriction

The skin is marked prior to the injection of a vasoconstrictor. The incision is placed 1.5 to 2 cm inferior to the mandible. Some surgeons place the incision parallel to the inferior border of the mandible; others place the incision in or parallel to a neck crease (see Fig. 9.3). Incisions made parallel to the inferior border of the mandible may be unobtrusive in some patients; however, extensions of this incision anteriorly may be noticeable unless hidden in the submandibular shadow. A less conspicuous scar results when the incision is made in or parallel to a skin crease. It should be noted that skin creases below the mandible do not parallel the inferior border of the mandible but run obliquely, posterosuperiorly to anteroinferiorly. Therefore, the further anterior the incision in or parallel to a skin crease, the more the distance to dissect to reach the inferior border of the mandible. Both incisions can be extended posteriorly to the mastoid region if necessary.

Mandibular fractures that shorten the vertical height of the ramus by their displacement (e.g., condylar fractures in patients without posterior teeth or those not placed into MMF) will cause the angle of the mandible to be more superior than it would be following reduction and fixation. Therefore, the incision should be placed 1.5 to 2 cm inferior to the *anticipated* location of the inferior border.

The incision is located along a suitable skin crease in the anteroposterior position that is needed for mandibular exposure. For a fracture that extends toward the gonial angle, the incision should begin behind and above the gonial angle, and extend downward and forward until it is in front of the gonial angle. For fractures located more anterior than the gonial angle, the incision does not have to extend behind and/or above the gonial angle, but may have to extend further anteriorly.

Vasoconstrictors with local anesthesia injected subcutaneously to aid hemostasis should not be placed deep to the platysma muscle because the marginal mandibular branch of the facial nerve may be rendered nonconductive, making electrical testing impossible. Alternatively, a vasoconstrictor without local anesthesia can be used both superficially and deep to the platysma muscle to promote hemostasis.

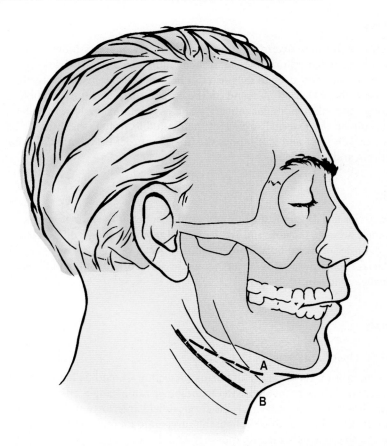

FIGURE 9.3 Two locations of submandibular incisions. Incision *A* parallels the inferior border of the mandible. Incision *B* parallels or is within the resting skin tension lines. Incision *B* leaves a less conspicuous scar in most patients.

➤ **STEP 3.** Skin Incision

The initial incision is carried through the skin and subcutaneous tissues to the level of the platysma muscle (see Fig. 9.4A). The skin is undermined with scissor dissection in all directions to facilitate closure. The superior portion of the incision is undermined approximately 1 cm; the inferior portion is undermined approximately 2 cm or more. The ends of the incision can be undermined extensively to allow retraction of the skin anteriorly or posteriorly to increase the extent of mandibular exposure. In this manner, a shorter skin incision can provide a large extent of exposure. Hemostasis is then achieved with electrocoagulation of bleeding subdermal vessels.

➤ **STEP 4.** Incising the Platysma Muscle

Retraction of the skin edges reveals the underlying platysma muscle, the fibers of which run superoinferiorly (Fig. 9.4B). Division of the fibers can be performed sharply, although a more controlled method is to dissect through the platysma muscle at one end of the skin incision with the tips of a hemostat or Metzenbaum scissors. After undermining the platysma muscle over the white superficial layer of deep cervical fascia, the tips of the instrument are pushed back through the platysma muscle at the other end of the incision. With the instrument deep to the platysma muscle, a scalpel is used to incise the muscle from one end of the skin incision to the other (see Fig. 9.5). The anterior and posterior skin edges can be retracted sequentially to allow a greater length of platysma muscle division than the length of the skin incision.

The platysma muscle passively contracts once divided, exposing the underlying superficial layer of deep cervical fascia (Fig. 9.5C). The submandibular salivary gland can also be visualized through the fascia, which helps form its capsule.

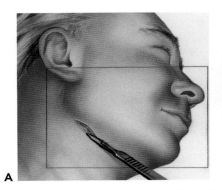
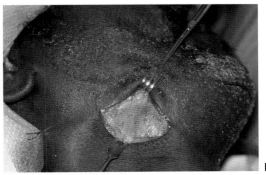

FIGURE 9.4 A: Incision through skin and subcutaneous tissue to the level of the platysma muscle. The incision parallels the lines of minimal tension in the cervical area. The incision does not parallel the inferior border of the mandible but courses inferiorly as it extends anteriorly. **B:** Photograph showing platysma muscle exposed by undermining of the skin and subcutaneous tissue.

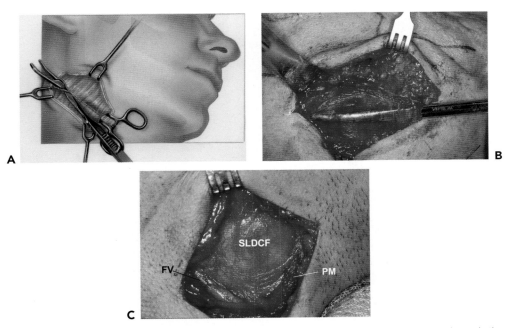

FIGURE 9.5 A: Illustration and **(B)**, photograph showing technique of sharp dissection through the platysma muscle that has been undermined with a hemostat. **C:** Photograph showing incised platysma muscle (*PM*) retracted and exposure of the superficial layer of deep cervical fascia overlying the submandibular gland (*SLDCF*). The facial vein can be seen at the posterior aspect of the incision, just deep to the platysma muscle (*FV*).

➤ **STEP 5.** Dissection to the Pterygomasseteric Muscular Sling

Dissection through the superficial layer of deep cervical fascia is the step that requires the most care because of the anatomic structures with which it is associated. The facial vein and artery are usually encountered when approaching the area of the premasseteric notch of the mandible, as well as the marginal mandibular branch of the facial nerve (see Fig. 9.6). The facial vessels can be isolated, clamped, divided, and ligated if they are intruding into the area

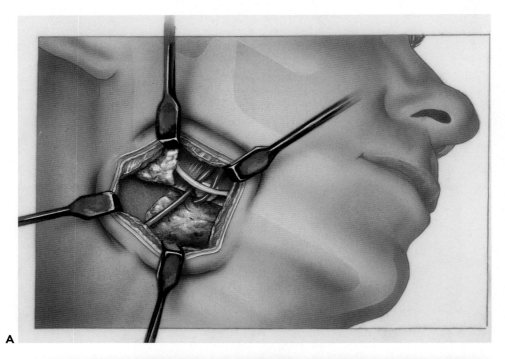

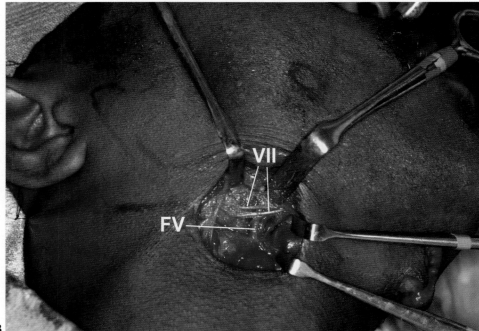

FIGURE 9.6 A: Illustration showing anatomic relation of the facial artery and vein, the marginal mandibular branch of the facial nerve, and the submandibular (premasseteric) lymph node to the inferior border of the mandible and masseter muscle. **B:** Photograph showing facial vessels (*FV*) and marginal mandibular branches of the facial nerve (*VII*).

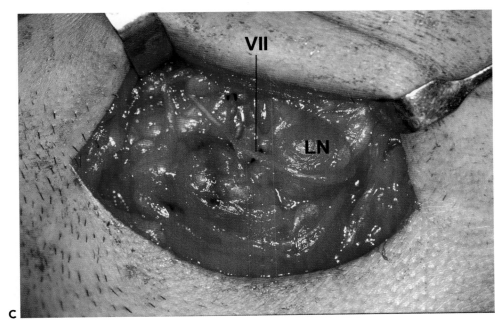

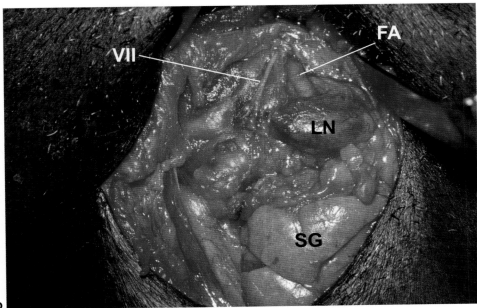

FIGURE 9.6 (*continued*) **C:** Photograph showing relation between marginal mandibular branch of the facial nerve (*VII*) and the submandibular lymph node (*LN*). **D:** Photograph showing relation of the submandibular lymph node (*LN*), the facial artery (*FA*), marginal mandibular branch of VII (*VII*) and the submandibular gland (*SG*).

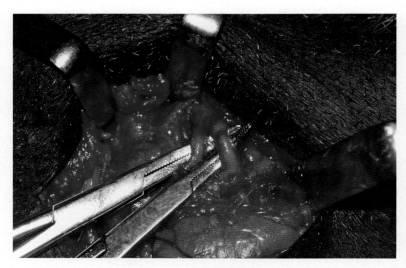

FIGURE 9.7 Photograph showing isolation of the facial artery and vein which can be ligated and divided.

of interest (see Fig. 9.7). When approaching the mandible posterior to the premasseteric notch, these vascular structures are not generally encountered; if they are, they are easily retracted anteriorly. However, care must be taken because the marginal mandibular branch is occasionally inferior to the mandible that is posterior to the premasseteric notch.

Dissection through the superficial layer of deep cervical fascia is accomplished by nicking it with a scalpel and undermining it bluntly with a hemostat or Metzenbaum scissors. The level of the incision and undermining of the fascia should be at least 1.5 cm inferior to the mandible to help protect the marginal mandibular branch of the facial nerve. Thus, dissection is performed *through* the fascia *at the level of the initial skin incision*, followed by dissection superiorly to the level of the periosteum of the mandible. The capsule of the submandibular salivary gland is often entered during this dissection, and the gland is retracted inferiorly (see Fig. 9.8). A consistent submandibular lymph node (Node of Stahr) is usually encountered in the area of the premasseteric notch and can be retracted superiorly or inferiorly. Its presence should alert the surgeon to the facial artery just anterior to the node, deep to the superficial layer of deep cervical fascia. The marginal mandibular branch of the facial nerve may be located close by, within or just deep to the superficial layer of deep cervical fascia, passing superficial to the facial vein and artery. An electrical nerve stimulator can be used to identify the nerve so that it can be retracted superiorly. In many instances, however, this facial nerve branch is located superior to the area of dissection and is not encountered.

Dissection continues until the only tissue remaining on the inferior border of the mandible is the periosteum (anterior to the premasseteric notch) or the pterygomasseteric sling (posterior to the premasseteric notch).

➤ STEP 6. Division of the Pterygomasseteric Sling and Submasseteric Dissection

With retraction of the dissected tissues superiorly and placement of a broad ribbon retractor just below the inferior border of the mandible to retract the submandibular tissues medially, the inferior border of the mandible is seen. The pterygomasseteric sling is sharply incised with a scalpel along the inferior border, which is the most avascular portion of the sling (see Fig. 9.9). Incisions in the lateral surface of the mandible into the masseter muscle often produce bothersome hemorrhage. Increased exposure of the mandible is possible by sequentially retracting the overlying tissues anteriorly and posteriorly, permitting more exposure of the inferior border for incision.

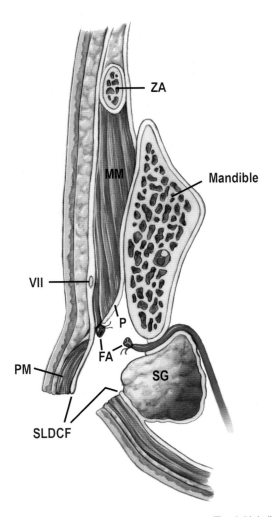

FIGURE 9.8 Coronal illustration showing the path of dissection. The initial dissection is through the platysma muscle (*PM*) to the superficial layer of deep cervical fascia (*SLDCF*), then through the area of the submandibular gland (*SG*) to the periosteum (*P*) of the mandible (*Mandible*), which is incised at the inferior border. *ZA*, zygomatic arch; *MM*, masseter muscle; *VII*, marginal mandibular branch of the facial nerve; *FA*, facial artery.

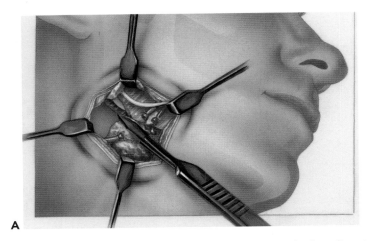

FIGURE 9.9 A: Illustration showing incision through the pterygomasseteric sling after retraction of vital structures. The incision should be at the inferior border of the mandible because it is the most avascular area in which the masseter and medial pterygoid muscles join.   (*continued*)

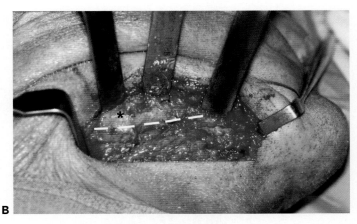

FIGURE 9.9 (*continued*) **B:** Photograph showing pterygomasseteric sling exposed (*) and line of incision inferior to the border of the mandible (*dashed line*).

The sharp end of a periosteal elevator is drawn along the length of the periosteal incision to strip the masseter muscle from the lateral ramus. Care is taken to keep the elevator in intimate contact with the bone, else shredding of the masseter results, causing bleeding and making retraction of the shredded tissue difficult. The entire lateral surface of the mandibular ramus (including the coronoid process) and body can be exposed to the level of the TMJ capsule (see Fig. 9.10), taking care to avoid perforating into the oral cavity along the retromolar area, if this is not desired. Once the buccinator muscle has been stripped from the retromolar area the only

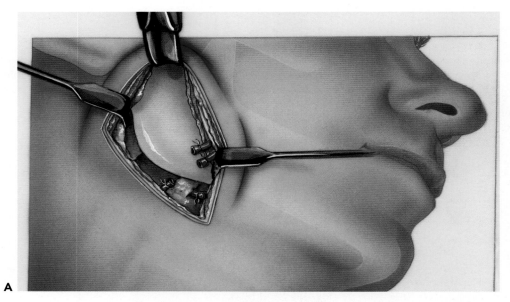

FIGURE 9.10 Illustration **(A)** demonstrating the extent of exposure obtained with the submandibular approach. The channel retractor is placed into the sigmoid notch, elevating the masseter, parotid, and superficial tissues. Exposure more anteriorly is accomplished by retraction in that direction.

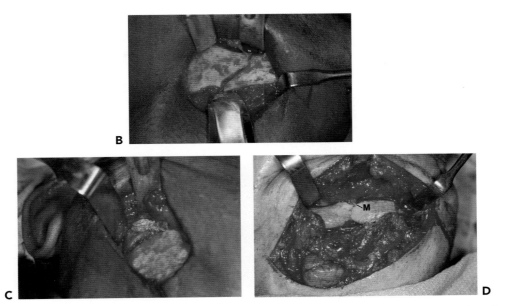

FIGURE 9.10 (*continued*) **B:** Photograph showing exposure in the area of the mandibular angle and body. **C:** Photograph showing exposure of the ramus and subcondylar regions (fractured). **D:** Photograph showing exposure of the mandibular body (fractured) and symphysis. The mental neurovascular bundle is clearly visible (*M*).

tissue separating the oral cavity from the dissection area is the oral mucosa. Retraction of the masseter muscle is facilitated by inserting a suitable retractor into the sigmoid notch (Channel retractor, Sigmoid notch retractor) (see Fig. 9.11).

More anterior in the mandibular body, care is needed to avoid damage to the mental neurovascular bundle (Fig. 9.10D), which exits the mental foramen, close to the apices of the bicuspid teeth.

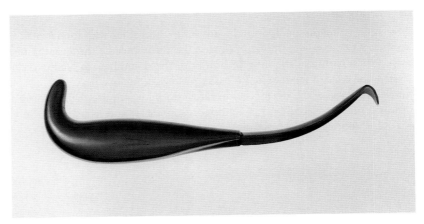

FIGURE 9.11 Sigmoid notch retractor. The curved flange inserts into the sigmoid notch, retracting the masseter muscle.

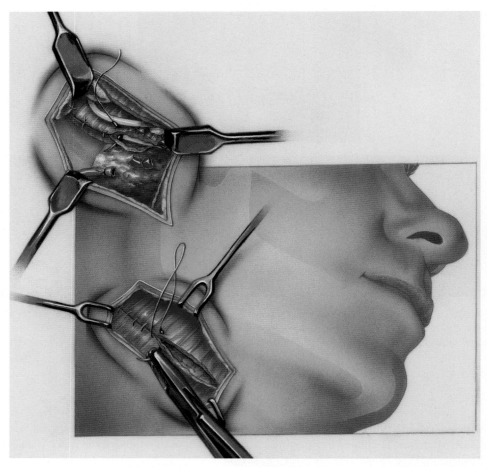

FIGURE 9.12 Closure of the pterygomasseteric sling (***inset***) and platysma. The pterygomasseteric sling is closed with resorbable interrupted suture. The platysma can be closed with a running resorbable suture, taking care to avoid damaging the underlying blood vessels and the seventh nerve.

➤ **STEP 7.** Closure

The masseter and medial pterygoid muscles are sutured together with interrupted resorbable sutures (see Fig. 9.12). It is often difficult to pass the suture needle through the medial pterygoid muscle which is thin at the inferior border of the mandible. To facilitate closure, it is possible to strip the edge of the muscle for easier passage of the needle.

The superficial layer of the deep cervical fascia does not require definitive suturing. The platysma muscle may be closed with a running resorbable suture (Fig. 9.12). Subcutaneous resorbable sutures followed by skin sutures are placed.

Extended Submandibular Approaches to the Inferior Border of the Mandible

Several choices are available if more exposure of the mandible becomes necessary. For increased ipsilateral exposure, the submandibular incision can be extended posteriorly toward the mastoid region, and anteriorly in an arcing manner toward the submental region (see Fig. 9.13). Once the incision leaves the direction of the resting skin tension lines however, the resultant scar will be more obvious.

To eliminate some of the undesirable scarring that may accompany the change in direction of the incision toward the submental area, one can step the anterior portion of the incision (see Fig. 9.14) (3).

Surgical splitting of the lower lip is another maneuver used occasionally in combination with incisions in the submandibular area to increase the exposure of one side of the mandible. It is possible to divide the lower lip in several ways. Each method uses the principle of breaking up the incision line to minimize scar contracture during healing (see Figs. 9.14 and 9.15).

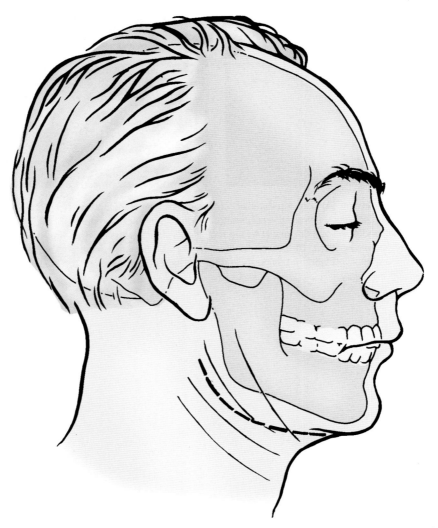

FIGURE 9.13 Extension of the submandibular incision posteriorly toward the mastoid region and anteriorly toward the submental region. Note that the incision leaves the resting skin tension lines anteriorly.

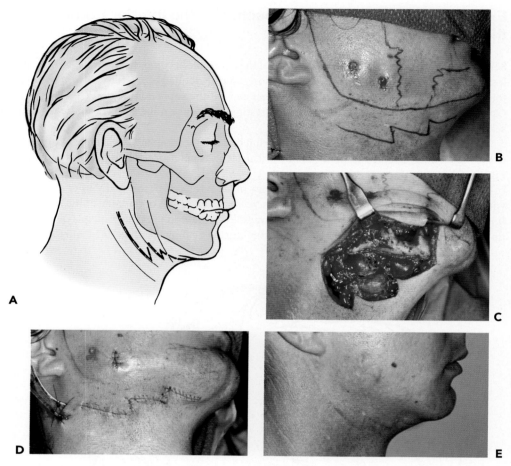

FIGURE 9.14 Illustration **(A)** showing extension of the submandibular incision posteriorly toward the mastoid region and anteriorly toward the submental region in a "stepped" manner. The longer arms of the steps should be kept close or parallel to the resting skin tension lines. Photographs showing the use of this incision in a patient. **B:** Incision marked on skin. **C:** Exposure of the mandible. Note the excellent exposure afforded without having to "tunnel" underneath the tissues. **D:** Closure of incision. **E:** Six weeks after surgery.

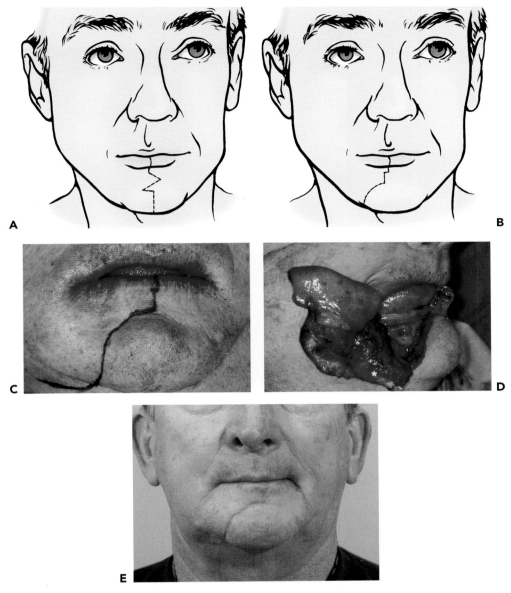

FIGURE 9.15 Two techniques of splitting the lower lip in the midline. These incisions can be connected to submandibular incisions on either side. **A:** Incision courses inferiorly through the genial soft tissue pad into the submental area. **B:** A technique of splitting the lip following the mentolabial crease. This technique is used in conjunction with a submandibular incision to increase exposure of that side of the mandible. **C:** Photograph showing lip-splitting incision on patient. **D:** Surgical photograph showing improved access provided by splitting the lip to remove mandibular specimen (*). **E:** Photograph 8 weeks after surgery.

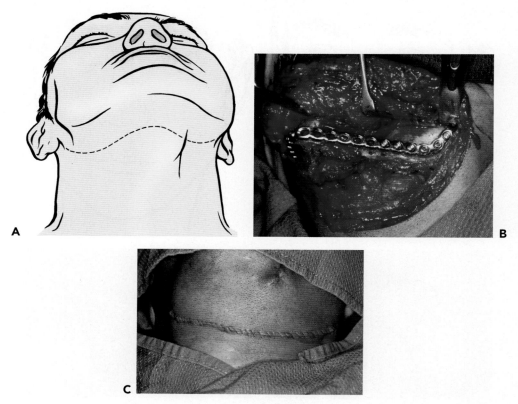

FIGURE 9.16 A: Illustration showing bilateral submandibular incisions connected in the midline for complete bilateral exposure of mandible. **B:** Photographs showing use of this incision for a large mandibular reconstruction, and after closure **(C)**.

For complete bilateral exposure of the mandible, one can use an "apron" flap with or without lip splitting. Bilateral submandibular incisions are extended into the neck and then connected. The incision may course somewhat toward the submental region or keep low in the neck, depending on the surgical requirements (see Fig. 9.16).

REFERENCES

1. Dingman RO, Grabb WC. Surgical anatomy of the mandibular ramus of the facial nerve based on the dissection of 100 facial halves. *Plast Reconstr Surg.* 1962;29:266.
2. Ziarah HA, Atkinson ME. The surgical anatomy of the cervical distribution of the facial nerve. *Br J Oral Maxillofac Surg.* 1981;19:159.
3. Zide M, Epker BN. An alternate elective neck incision. *J Oral Maxillofac Surg.* 1993;51:1071.

10

Retromandibular Approach

The retromandibular approach exposes the entire ramus from behind the posterior border. It therefore may be useful for procedures involving the area on or near the condylar neck/head, or the ramus itself. In this approach the distance from the skin incision to the area of interest is reduced compared to that of the submandibular approach.

Surgical Anatomy

Facial Nerve

The main trunk of the facial nerve emerges from the skull base at the stylomastoid foramen. It lies medial, deep, and slightly anterior to the middle of the mastoid process at the lower end of the tympanomastoid fissure. After giving off the posterior auricular and branches to the posterior digastric and stylohyoid muscles, it passes obliquely inferiorly and laterally into the substance of the parotid gland. The length of the facial nerve trunk that is visible to the surgeon is approximately 1.3 cm. It divides into the temporofacial and cervicofacial divisions at a point vertically below the lowest part of the bony external auditory meatus (see Fig. 10.1).

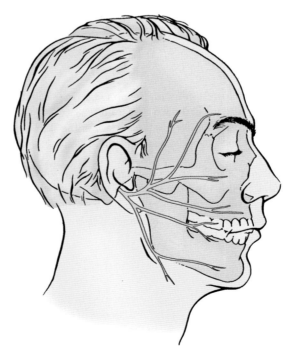

FIGURE 10.1 Branching of the extracranial portion of the facial nerve. Only the main branches are shown. Many smaller branches occur in most individuals (Fig. 10.2).

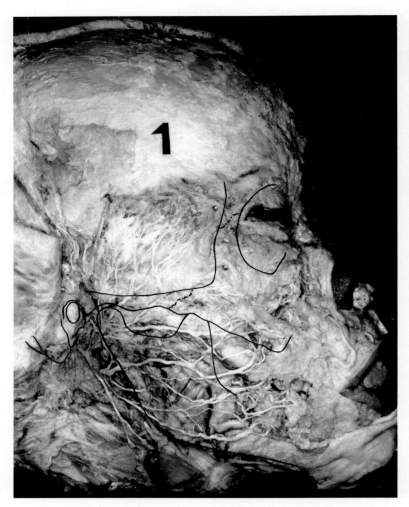

FIGURE 10.2 Anatomic dissection reveals an extensive branching pattern of the facial nerve (the parotid gland was removed).

The average distance from the lowest point on the bony external auditory meatus to the bifurcation of the facial nerve is 2.3 cm (Standard deviation 0.28 cm) (1). Posterior to the parotid gland, the nerve trunk is at least 2 cm deep to the surface of the skin. Its two divisions proceed forward in the substance of the parotid gland and divide into their terminal branches (see Fig. 10.2).

The marginal mandibular branch courses obliquely and anteriorly downward. It frequently rises from the main trunk well behind the posterior border of the mandible and crosses the posterior border in the lower one third of the ramus. This positioning leaves a void between the buccal branches and the marginal mandibular branch or branches through which the mandible can be approached safely (see Fig. 10.3).

Retromandibular Vein

The retromandibular vein (posterior facial vein) is formed in the upper portion of the parotid gland, deep to the neck of the mandible, by the confluence of the superficial temporal vein and the maxillary vein. Descending just posterior to the ramus of the mandible through the parotid gland, or folded into its deep aspect, the vein is lateral to the external carotid artery (Fig. 10.3). Both vessels are crossed by the facial nerve. Near the apex of the parotid gland, the retromandibular vein gives off an anteriorly descending communication that joins the facial vein just

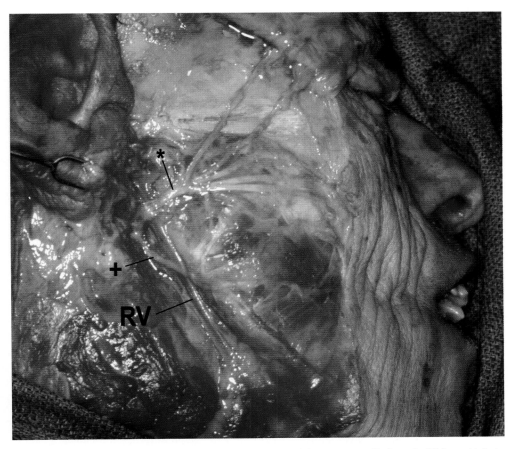

FIGURE 10.3 Anatomic dissection showing the relation of the retromandibular vein (*RV*), and inferior (+) and superior divisions (*) of nerve VII to the mandible. Note the space between the inferior and superior divisions of nerve VII, through which the posterior border of the mandible can be approached.

below the angle of the mandible. The retromandibular vein then inclines backward and unites with the posterior auricular vein to form the external jugular vein.

Technique

The position of the skin incision, which also dictates the position of the underlying dissection, varies in the retromandibular approach to the mandible. Some surgeons advocate placing of an incision approximately 2 cm posterior to the ramus. The parotid gland is approached from behind and sharply dissected from the sternocleidomastoid muscle, allowing retraction of the gland superiorly and anteriorly to gain access to the ramus. The theoretic advantage of this approach is that it avoids the branching facial nerve, which is contained within the parotid gland. Unfortunately, the primary advantage of the retromandibular approach, which is the direct proximity of the skin incision to the mandible, is then lost. An alternate approach that was described by Hinds (2) is described in this chapter. The incision is placed along the posterior border of the mandible, just below the earlobe. Dissection to the posterior border of the mandible is direct, traversing the parotid gland, and exposing some branches of the facial nerve (Video 10.1).

➤ **STEP 1.** Preparation and Draping

Pertinent landmarks of the face such as the corner of the mouth, lower lip, and the entire ear should be left uncovered during the procedure (see Fig. 10.4). These landmarks orient the surgeon to the course of the facial nerve and allow observation of lip motor function.

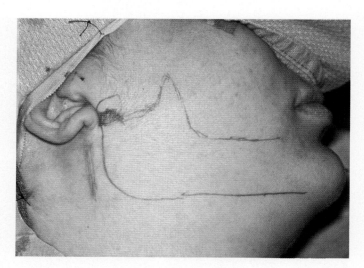

FIGURE 10.4 Photograph of patient draped and marked for surgery.

➤ **STEP 2.** Marking the Incision and Vasoconstriction

The skin is marked prior to the injection of a vasoconstrictor. The incision for the retromandibular approach begins 0.5 cm below the earlobe and continues inferiorly for 3 to 3.5 cm (see Figs. 10.4 and 10.5). It is placed just behind the posterior border of the mandible and may or may not extend below the level of the mandibular angle, depending on the extent of exposure desired.

Epinephrine (1:200,000) without a local anesthetic may be injected deeply, although routine local anesthetics with a vasoconstrictor should be injected only subcutaneously to aid in hemostasis at the time of incision. Even though the facial nerve is located deeper than 2 cm at the earlobe, injection of local anesthetics deep to the platysma muscle risks rendering the facial nerve branches nonconductive, making electrical testing impossible.

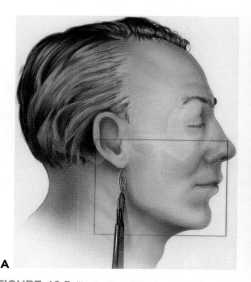

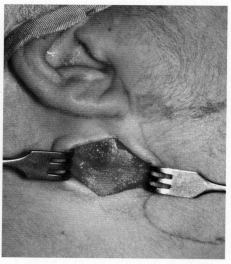

A

B

FIGURE 10.5 Illustration **(A)** showing placement of vertical incision just posterior to the mandible through skin and subcutaneous tissue to the depth of the platysma muscle. **B:** Photograph showing scant platysma muscle and underlying superficial musculoaponeurotic system (SMAS) after the skin has been incised and undermined.

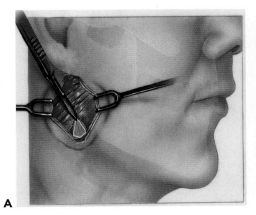
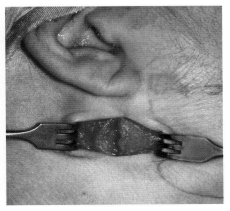

FIGURE 10.6 A: Illustration showing incision through platysma, superficial musculoaponeurotic system (SMAS), and parotid fascia into substance of gland. **B:** Photograph after incision into parotid gland demonstrating glandular tissue entered.

➤ STEP 3. Skin Incision

The initial incision is carried through skin and subcutaneous tissues to the level of the scant platysma muscle present in this area. Undermining the skin with scissors in all directions allows ease of retraction and facilitates closure (Fig. 10.5B). Hemostasis is then achieved with electrocoagulation of bleeding subdermal vessels.

➤ STEP 4. Dissection to the Pterygomasseteric Muscular Sling

After retraction of the skin edges, the scant platysma muscle overlying the superficial musculoaponeurotic system (SMAS) is visible. A scalpel is used to incise through the fusion of platysma muscle, SMAS, and parotid capsule in the vertical plane. The gland will be clearly visible once entered (see Fig. 10.6). Blunt dissection begins within the gland in an anteromedial direction toward the posterior border of the mandible. A hemostat is spread open parallel to the anticipated direction of the facial nerve branches (see Fig. 10.7). The marginal mandibular branch of the facial nerve is often, but not always, encountered during this dissection and may be intentionally sought with a nerve stimulator (see Fig. 10.8). The cervical branch of the facial nerve may also be encountered, but it is of little consequence as it runs vertically out of the field (see Fig. 10.9). In many instances, the marginal mandibular branch interferes with exposure and may be retracted superiorly or inferiorly depending on its location. A useful adjunct in retracting the marginal mandibular branch involves dissecting it free from surrounding tissues proximally for 1 cm and distally for 1.5 to 2 cm. This simple maneuver will help determine whether it is better to retract the nerve superiorly or inferiorly. Dissection then continues until the only tissue remaining on the posterior border of the mandible is the periosteum of

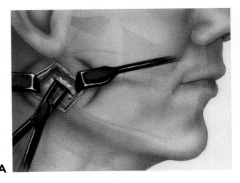
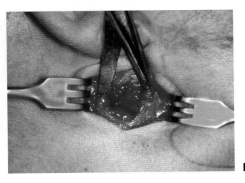

FIGURE 10.7 A: Illustration and **(B)**, photograph showing blunt dissection through the parotid gland, spreading the hemostat in the direction of the fibers of VII.

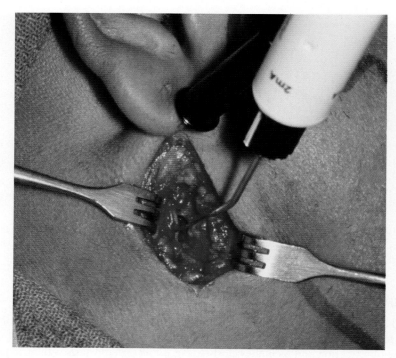

FIGURE 10.8 Photograph showing use of a nerve stimulator to identify branches of the facial nerve.

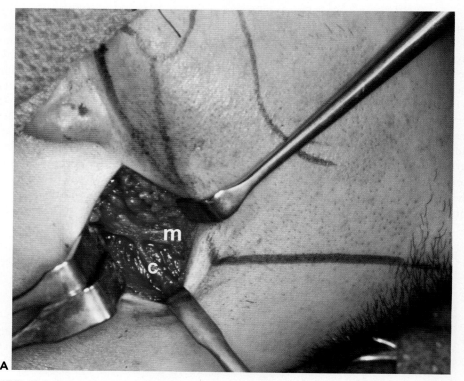

FIGURE 10.9 Examples of the variation in facial nerve anatomy. **A:** Three branches of the marginal mandibular nerve are shown coursing anteriorly (*m*) while the cervical branch is shown coursing inferiorly (*c*).

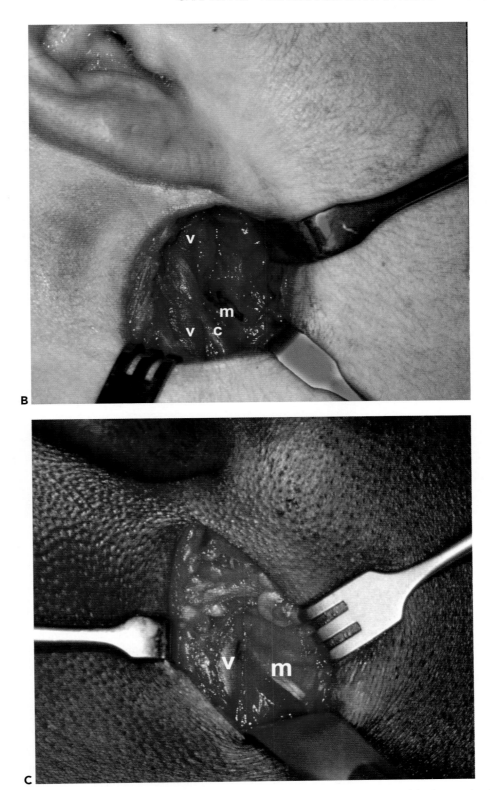

FIGURE 10.9 (*continued*) **B:** Marginal mandibular (*m*) and cervical branches (*c*) shown closely adapted to the lateral surface of the retromandibular vein (*v*) **C:** In this photograph, the marginal mandibular branch (*m*) is seen coursing deep to the retromandibular vein (*v*).

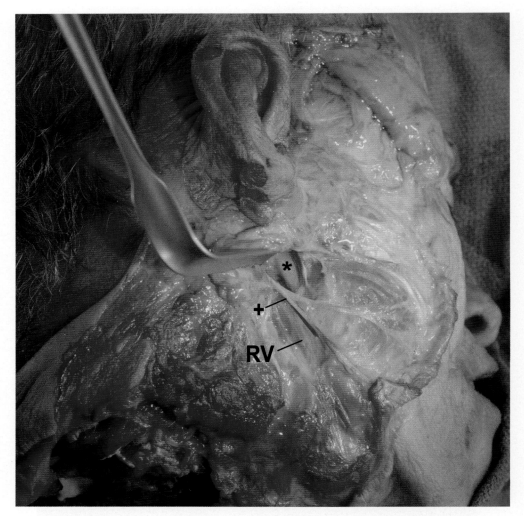

FIGURE 10.10 The surgical window to the posterior mandible is revealed by retraction of tissues between inferior (+) and superior divisions of VII. The retractor is on the neck of the condyle (*). Note the path of the retromandibular vein (*RV*). The inferior division of VII can be retracted further inferiorly to allow access to the gonial angle.

the pterygomasseteric sling (see Fig. 10.10). One should also be aware of the retromandibular vein, which runs vertically in the same plane of dissection and is commonly exposed along its entire retromandibular course. This vein rarely requires ligation unless it has been inadvertently transected.

➤ **STEP 5.** Division of the Pterygomasseteric Sling and Submasseteric Dissection

After retraction of the dissected tissues anteriorly (with the marginal mandibular branch of the facial nerve perhaps under the retractor), a broad retractor such as a ribbon retractor is placed behind the posterior border of the mandible to retract the retromandibular tissues medially. The posterior border of the mandible with the overlying pterygomasseteric sling is seen (see Fig. 10.11A). The pterygomasseteric sling is incised sharply with a scalpel (Fig. 10.11B). The incision begins as far superiorly as reachable and extends as far inferiorly around the gonial angle as possible. An incision placed in the posterior portion of the sling bleeds less than an incision placed more laterally through the belly of the masseter muscle.

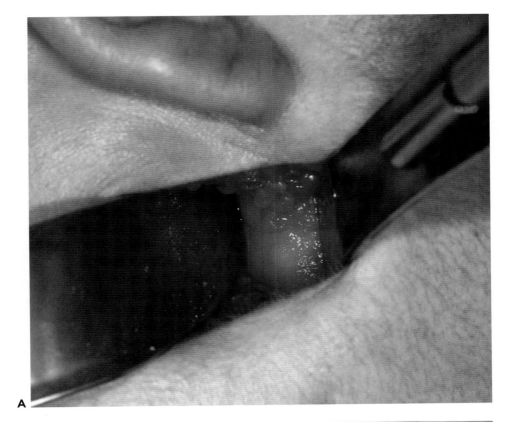

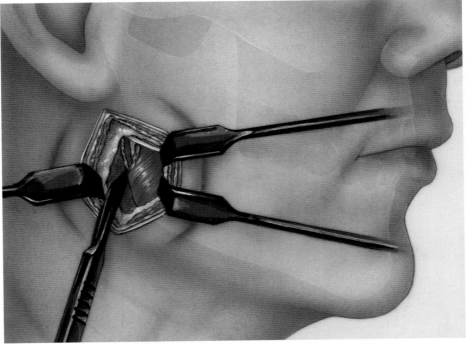

FIGURE 10.11 A: Photograph showing exposure of the posterior border of the mandibular ramus after dissection through the parotid gland. Retractors on the medial and lateral surface of the ramus provide exposure of the pterygomasseteric sling, which is clearly shown here prior to incision. **B:** Illustration showing incision through the pterygomasseteric sling along the posterior border of the mandible. The inferior division of VII is being retracted superiorly in this example, but often is retracted inferiorly and exposure is between the buccal branches above and the marginal mandibular branch(es) below.

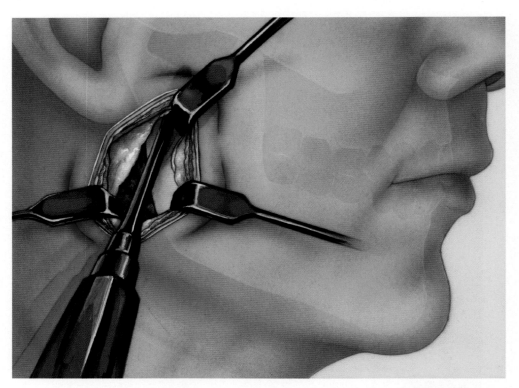

FIGURE 10.12 Subperiosteal dissection of the masseter muscle. The periosteal elevator is used to strip the muscle fibers from top to bottom of the ramus.

The sharp end of a periosteal elevator is drawn along the length of the incision to strip the tissues from the posterior border of the ramus. The masseter is stripped from the lateral surface of the mandible using periosteal elevators. Clean dissection is facilitated by stripping the muscle from top to bottom (see Fig. 10.12). Keeping the elevator in intimate contact with the bone reduces shredding and bleeding of the masseter. The entire lateral surface of the mandibular ramus, up to the level of the temporomandibular joint capsule as well as the coronoid process, can be exposed. Retraction of the masseter muscle is facilitated by inserting a suitable retractor into the sigmoid notch (e.g., Channel retractor, Sigmoid notch retractor) (see Figs. 10.13, 10.14, and 10.15).

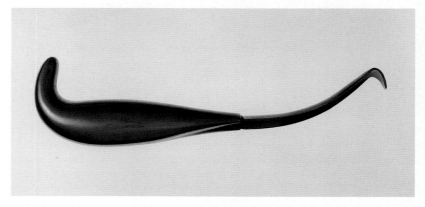

FIGURE 10.13 Sigmoid notch retractor. The curved flange at the end is inserted into the sigmoid notch, retracting the masseter muscle.

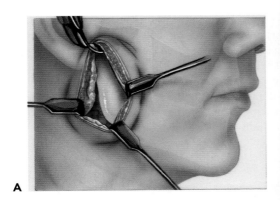
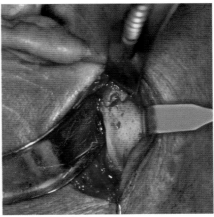

FIGURE 10.14 Illustration **(A)** and photograph **(B)** showing exposure of the posterior ramus. The sigmoid notch retractor is placed into the sigmoid notch, elevating the masseter, parotid, and superficial tissues.

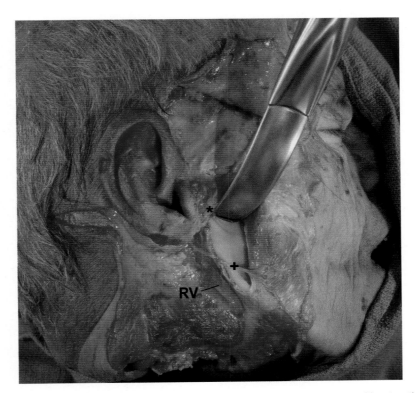

FIGURE 10.15 Anatomic dissection showing exposure of the posterior ramus with retraction of the superior division of VII by the channel retractor (*). +, marginal mandibular branch VII; *RV*, retromandibular vein.

When using this approach for open treatment of condylar process fractures, it is often necessary to distract the mandibular ramus inferiorly. A simple technique to do this is by first applying a bicortical bone screw through the gonial angle region, taking care to avoid the inferior alveolar canal (see Fig. 10.16A). A 14-gauge needle is passed through the skin below the angle of the mandible and into the surgical field (Fig. 10.16B). The closed end of a 24-gauge wire loop is passed through the needle (Fig. 10.16C) and retrieved from within the surgical field. The needle is withdrawn leaving only the wires exiting the skin. The loop is placed over the bone screw and the wires are twisted, securing the wire to the bone screw (Fig. 10.16D). A wire twister can then be used to pull the wires and the mandible inferiorly.

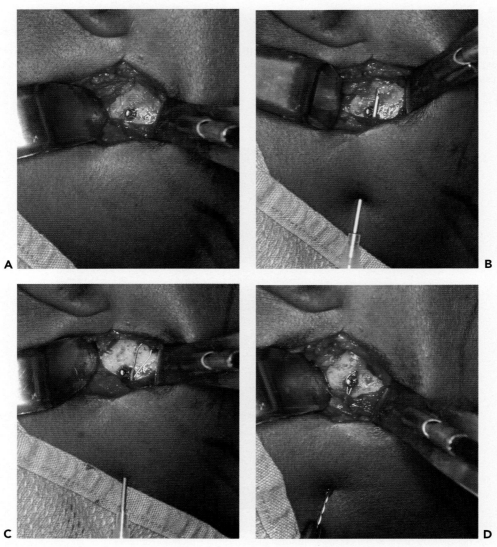

FIGURE 10.16 Photographs showing the method of placing a traction wire that can be used to distract the gonial angle inferiorly. **A:** One bicortical screw placed through mandible. **B:** Needle inserted through skin into surgical field **C:** Loop of 24-gauge wire inserted through needle. **D:** Wire placed around bone screw and ends of wire twisted together.

➤ **STEP 6.** Closure

The masseter and medial pterygoid muscles are sutured together with interrupted resorbable sutures. It may be difficult to pass the suture needle through the medial pterygoid muscle which is very thin at the inferior and posterior borders of the mandible. To facilitate closure, the suture should first be passed through the masseter muscle (see Fig. 10.17A). The edge of the medial pterygoid muscle can be stripped a few millimeters for easier needle passage. However, another way to facilitate passing the suture through the edge of the medial pterygoid muscle is to pass the needle in the sagittal plane, deep to, but up against, the mandible (Fig. 10.17B). This first suture may be delayed until another is placed. Typically, only two sutures are necessary to reapproximate the pterygomasseteric sling along the posterior border (Fig. 10.17C) unless the sling below the angle of the mandible has been incised. In that case, sutures must also be placed through the sling along the inferior border of the mandible.

Closure of the parotid capsule/SMAS and platysma layer is important to avoid a salivary fistula. A running, slowly resorbing horizontal mattress suture is used to tightly close the parotid capsule, SMAS, and the platysma muscle in one watertight layer (see Fig. 10.18). Placement of subcutaneous sutures is followed by skin closure.

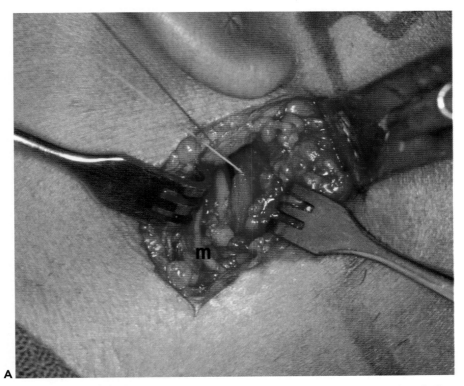

FIGURE 10.17 Photographs showing a method of suturing the pterygomasseteric sling. **A:** Suture is passed through the masseter muscle. Note the position of the marginal mandibular branch of the facial nerve (*m*). *(continued)*

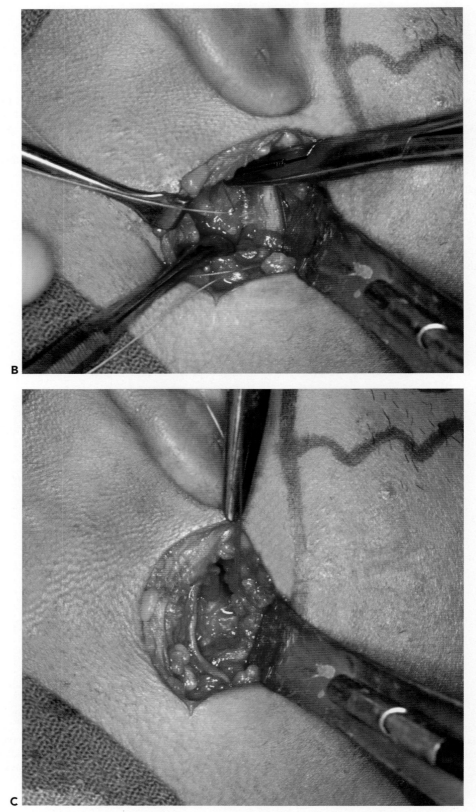

FIGURE 10.17 (*continued*) **B:** Suture needle passing through the medial pterygoid muscle on the medial aspect of the mandible. **C:** Suture tied, reapproximating pterygomasseteric sling.

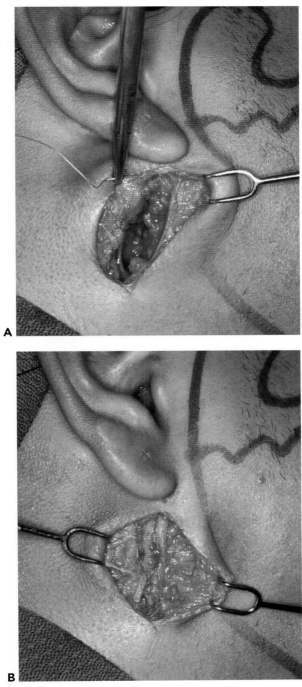

FIGURE 10.18 Photographs showing closure of the parotid capsule/superficial musculoaponeurotic system (SMAS)/platysma muscle. **A:** Suture is passed through these fused layers on one side of the incision. **B:** Closure after a running horizontal mattress suture has been placed. Notice the eversion of these layers and the watertight closure.

Alternative Approaches to the Mandibular Ramus

Additional exposure of the mandibular ramus is frequently required. Combinations of approaches such as the preauricular approach and the retromandibular approach offer increased exposure for some procedures, such as those for temporomandibular ankylosis. If even greater exposure is required, these two approaches can be connected, using a modified Blair incision (see Fig. 10.19). This incision is used frequently for surgeries involving the parotid gland, but it is also useful for those involving the mandibular ramus.

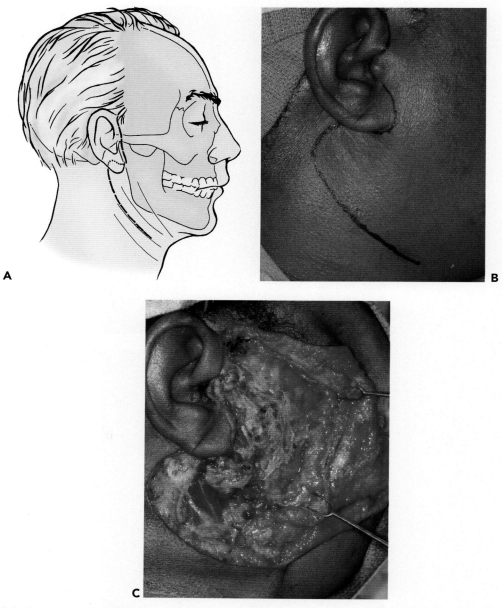

FIGURE 10.19 Modified Blair incision. The preauricular and retromandibular approaches are connected by an incision hidden in the lobular crease of the ear. The anteroposterior position of the retromandibular portion of the approach may be customized. In this illustration **(A)**, the incision parallels the sternocleidomastoid muscle and is more posterior than the retromandibular approach described previously. In these clinical photos **(B** and **C)**, the incision combines components of the preauricular, retromandibular, and submandibular approaches.

REFERENCES

1. Al-Kayat A, Bramley P. A modified pre-auricular approach to the temporomandibular joint and malar arch. *Br J Oral Maxillofac Surg.* 1979;17:91.
2. Hinds EC. Correction of prognathism by subcondylar osteotomy. *J Oral Maxillofac Surg.* 1958;16:209.

11

Rhytidectomy Approach

The rhytidectomy or facelift approach to the mandibular ramus is a variant of the retromandibular approach. The only difference is that the cutaneous incision is placed in a more hidden location as in a facelift. The procedure for the deeper dissection is the same as that described for the retromandibular approach.

The main advantage of the rhytidectomy approach to the ramus is the less conspicuous facial scar. The disadvantage is the additional time required for closure.

Surgical Anatomy

Great Auricular Nerve

The only significant structure specific to this approach, not mentioned for the retromandibular approach, is the great auricular nerve. This sensory nerve begins deep in the neck as spinal roots C2 and C3, which fuse on the scalene muscles to form the great auricular nerve. As the nerve becomes more superficial, it emerges through the deep fascia of the neck at the middle of the posterior border of the sternocleidomastoid muscle. It crosses the sternocleidomastoid muscle at a 45-degree angle to the mandible, covered only by the superficial musculoaponeurotic system (SMAS) and the skin, and lies behind the external jugular vein. The nerve then may split into two branches as it courses superiorly toward the earlobe (see Fig. 11.1). Some branches pass through the parotid gland and supply the skin of a part of the outer ear and a variably wide area in the mandibular angle region.

Technique

➤ **STEP 1.** Preparation and Draping

Pertinent landmarks on the face useful during dissection should be exposed throughout the surgical procedure. When using the rhytidectomy approach to the mandibular ramus/angle, the structures that should be visible in the field include the corner of the eye, the corner of the mouth, and the lower lip anteriorly, and the entire ear and descending hairline, and 2 to 3 cm of hair superior to the posterior hairline, posteriorly. The temporal area must also be completely exposed. Inferiorly, several centimeters of skin below the inferior border of the mandible are exposed to provide access for undermining the skin. Shaving the sideburns and temporal hair is unnecessary, except from a convenience standpoint.

➤ **STEP 2.** Marking the Incision and Vasoconstriction

The skin is marked before injecting a vasoconstrictor. The incision begins approximately 1.5 to 2 cm superior to the zygomatic arch just posterior to the anterior extent of the hairline

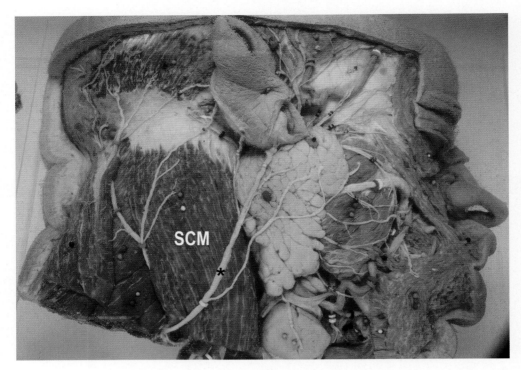

FIGURE 11.1 Anatomic dissection showing the relation of the great auricular nerve (*) to the sterno-cleidomastoid muscle (*SCM*) and ear.

(see Fig. 11.2). The incision then curves posteriorly and inferiorly, blending into a preauricular incision in the natural crease anterior to the pinna (the same position as in the preauricular approach to the temporomandibular joint). The incision continues under the earlobe and approximately 3 mm onto the posterior surface of the auricle instead of continuing in the mastoid–ear skin crease. This modification prevents a noticeable scar that occurs during contractive healing of the flap, pulling the scar into the neck; instead, the scar ends in the crease between the auricle and the mastoid skin. At a point where the incision is well hidden by the ear, it curves posteriorly toward the hairline and then runs along the hairline, or just inside it, for a few centimeters.

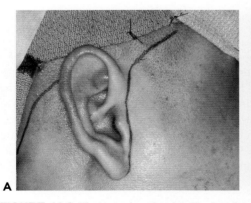
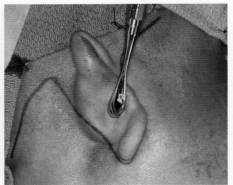

FIGURE 11.2 Photographs showing the location of the incision in a male patient. **A:** The incision can be extended forward into the hairline for better retraction. **B:** The incision extends to the posterior aspect of the ear before sweeping down the hairline.

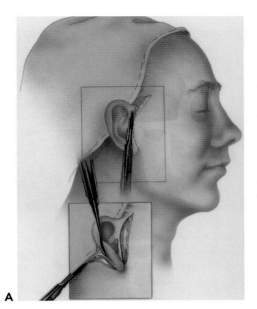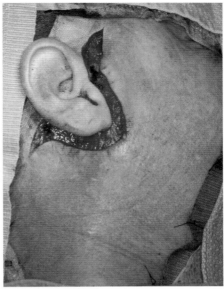

FIGURE 11.3 **A:** Illustration demonstrating incision through skin and subcutaneous tissue. **B:** Photograph of a female patient showing incision and dissection into the subcutaneous layer.

A vasoconstrictor is injected subcutaneously to aid in hemostasis at the time of incision. Local anesthetics should not be injected deep to the platysma muscle because of the risk of rendering the facial nerve branches nonconductive, making electrical testing impossible.

➤ **STEP 3.** Skin Incision and Dissection

The initial incision is made through the skin and subcutaneous tissue only (see Fig. 11.3). A skin flap is elevated through this incision using sharp and blunt dissection with Metzenbaum or rhytidectomy scissors (see Fig. 11.4). The flap should be widely undermined to create a subcutaneous pocket that extends below the angle of the mandible and a few centimeters

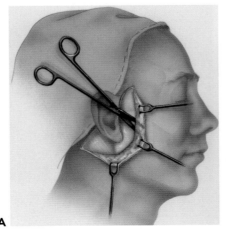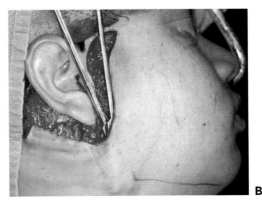

FIGURE 11.4 Illustration **(A)** and photograph **(B)** showing undermining of the skin with Metzenbaum or facelift scissors.

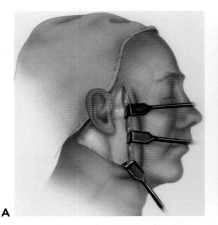
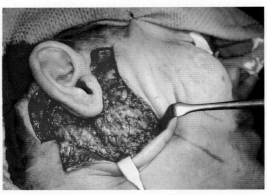

FIGURE 11.5 Illustration **(A)** and photograph **(B)** showing the extent of subcutaneous dissection necessary for exposing the posterior mandible. The skin should be completely freed so that it can be retracted below the angle of the mandible and to the premasseteric notch.

anterior to the posterior border of the mandible. There are no anatomic structures of any significance in this plane except for the great auricular nerve, which is deep to the subcutaneous dissection. Hemostasis is then achieved with electrocoagulation of the bleeding subdermal vessels.

➤ **STEP 4.** Retromandibular Approach

Once the skin has been retracted anteriorly and inferiorly, the soft tissues overlying the posterior half of the mandibular ramus are visible (see Fig. 11.5). From this point onward, the dissection proceeds exactly as described for the retromandibular approach. The bony access is the same in both approaches (see Fig. 11.6).

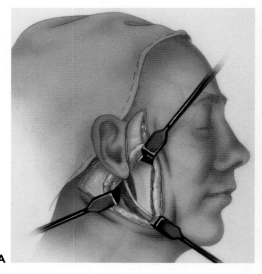
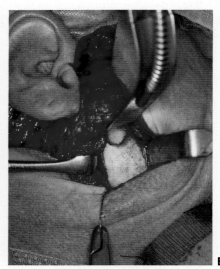

FIGURE 11.6 Illustration **(A)** and photograph **(B)** showing the posterior mandible exposed through the rhytidectomy approach. A condylar neck fracture is being approached in this clinical photograph. The retractors are used to retract the masseter, parotid, and superior branches of cranial nerve VII.

➤ **STEP 5.** Closure

Deep closure is performed as described for the retromandibular approach. After the parotid capsule/SMAS/platysma layer is closed, a 1/8- or 3/32-inch round vacuum drain is placed into the subcutaneous pocket to prevent hematoma formation. The drain can exit the posterior portion of the incision or through a separate stab in the posterior part of the neck. A two-layer skin closure is performed (see Fig. 11.7).

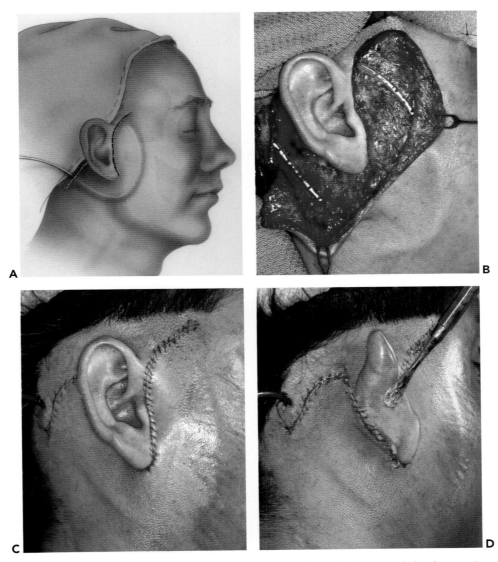

FIGURE 11.7 Illustration **(A)** and photographs **(B–D)** showing subcutaneous drain placement and closure.

SECTION 6

Approaches to the Temporomandibular Joint

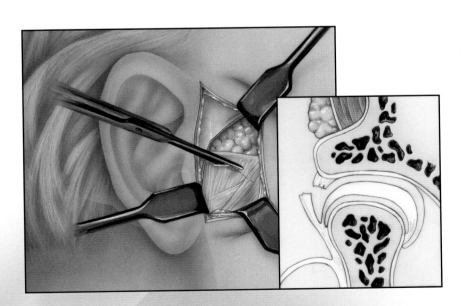

The temporomandibular joint (TMJ) and its components frequently require exposure for a myriad of procedures. Internal derangements of the TMJ, arthritis, trauma, developmental disorders, and neoplasia may all affect the TMJ and/or the skeletal and soft tissue components. Several approaches to the TMJ have been proposed and used clinically. The standard and most basic approach, however, is the preauricular approach, which is described in detail in this section. Variations are briefly mentioned.

12 Preauricular Approach

The temporomandibular joint (TMJ) is situated in an area that is relatively easy to expose surgically, although the extent of exposure obtained is not much. The structure that limits the extent of exposure is the branching facial nerve.

Surgical Anatomy

Although the TMJ itself is relatively small, there are many important anatomic structures near it. This region contains the parotid gland, superficial temporal vessels, and facial and auriculotemporal nerves.

Parotid Gland

The parotid gland lies below the zygomatic arch, below and in front of the external acoustic meatus, on the masseter muscle, and behind the ramus of the mandible. The superficial pole of the parotid gland lies directly on the TMJ capsule. The parotid gland itself is enclosed within a capsule derived from the superficial layer of the deep cervical fascia, frequently called the *parotideomasseteric fascia*.

Superficial Temporal Vessels

The superficial temporal vessels emerge from the superior aspect of the parotid gland and accompany the auriculotemporal nerve (see Fig. 12.1). The superficial temporal artery rises in the parotid gland by bifurcation of the external carotid artery (the other terminal artery is the internal maxillary). As it crosses superficial to the zygomatic arch, a temporal branch is given off just over the arch. This vessel is a common source of bleeding during surgery. The superficial temporal artery divides into the frontal and parietal branches a few centimeters above the arch. The superficial temporal vein lies superficial and usually posterior to the artery. The auriculotemporal nerve accompanies, and is posterior to, the superficial temporal artery.

Auriculotemporal Nerve

The auriculotemporal nerve innervates parts of the auricle, the external auditory meatus, the tympanic membrane, and the skin in the temporal area. It courses from the medial side of the posterior neck of the condyle and turns superiorly, running over the zygomatic root of the temporal bone (Fig. 12.1). Just anterior to the auricle, the nerve divides into its terminal branches in the skin of the temporal area. Preauricular exposure of the TMJ area almost

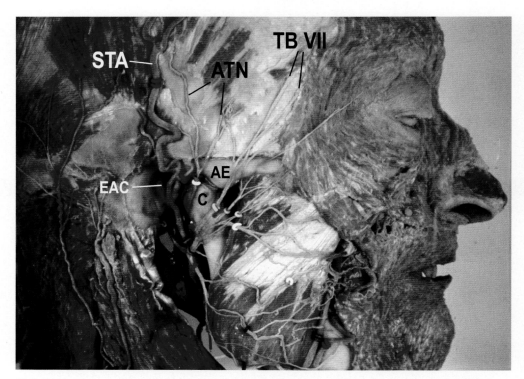

FIGURE 12.1 Anatomic dissection showing structures of importance. *C*, condyle; *AE*, articular eminence of the temporal bone; *EAC*, external auditory canal (outer ear removed); *STA*, superficial temporal artery; *ATN*, auriculotemporal nerves; *TB VII*, temporal branches of the facial nerve.

invariably injures this nerve. The damage is minimized by incising and dissecting in close apposition to the cartilaginous portion of the external auditory meatus, realizing that this structure runs somewhat anteriorly as it courses from lateral to medial. Temporal extension of the skin incision should be located posteriorly so that the main distribution of the nerve is dissected and retracted forward within the flap. Fortunately, patients rarely complain about sensory disturbances that result from damage to this nerve.

Facial Nerve

Shortly after the facial nerve exits the skull through the stylomastoid foramen, it enters the parotid gland. At this point, the nerve usually divides into two main trunks (temporofacial and cervicofacial), the branches of which variably anastomose to form a parotid plexus. The division of the facial nerve is located between 1.5 and 2.8 cm below the lowest concavity of the bony external auditory canal.

The terminal branches of the facial nerve emerge from the parotid gland and radiate anteriorly (Fig. 12.1). They are commonly classified as temporal, zygomatic, buccal, marginal mandibular, and cervical. The location of the temporal branches is of particular concern during TMJ surgery because these are the branches that are most likely to be damaged. As the temporal nerve branches (frequently two) cross the lateral surface of the zygomatic arch, they course along the undersurface of the temporoparietal fascia (see Fig. 6.5). The temporal branch crosses the zygomatic arch at varying locations in different individuals, and may be located anywhere from 8 to 35 mm (20 mm average) anterior to the external auditory canal (see Fig. 12.2) (1). Therefore, the temporal branches of the facial nerve can be protected by incising through the

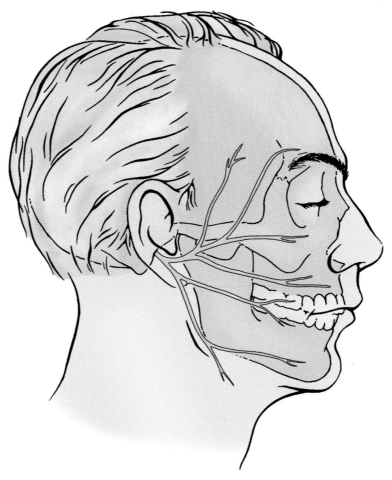

FIGURE 12.2 Major branches of the facial nerve. The distance from the anterior concavity of the external auditory canal to the crossing of the zygomatic arch by the temporal branch varies from 8 to 35 mm.

superficial layer of temporalis fascia and periosteum of the zygomatic arch not more than 0.8 cm in front of the anterior border of the external auditory canal.

Temporomandibular Joint

The TMJ capsule defines the anatomic and functional boundaries of the TMJ. The thin, loose fibrous capsule surrounds the articular surface of the condyle and blends with the periosteum of the mandibular neck. On the temporal bone, the articular capsule completely surrounds the articular surfaces of the eminence and fossa (see Fig. 12.3). The attachments of the capsule are firmly adhered to the bone. Anteriorly, the capsule attaches in front of the crest of the articular eminence; laterally, it adheres to the edge of the eminence and fossa; and posteriorly, it extends medially along the anterior lip of the squamotympanic and petrotympanic fissures. The medial attachment runs along the sphenosquamosal suture. The articular capsule is strongly reinforced laterally by the temporomandibular (lateral) ligament, composed of a superficial fan-shaped layer of obliquely oriented connective tissue fibers and a deeper, narrow band of fibers that run more horizontally. The ligament attaches broadly to the outer surface of the root of the zygomatic arch and converges downward and backward to attach to the back of the condyle below and behind its lateral pole.

The articular disk is a firm but flexible structure with a biconcave shape (see Fig. 12.4). The disk is usually divided into three regions: the posterior band, the intermediate zone, and the anterior band. The central intermediate zone is considerably thinner (1 mm) than the posterior (3 mm) and anterior (2 mm) bands. The upper surface of the disk adapts to the contours

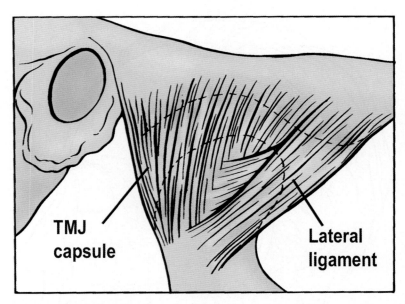

FIGURE 12.3 The temporomandibular joint (*TMJ*) capsule and lateral ligament. The lateral ligament has both oblique and horizontal components.

of the fossa and the eminence of the temporal bone, and the lower surface of the disk adapts to the contour of the mandibular condyle.

Posteriorly, the disk and the loosely organized posterior attachment tissues (i.e., bilaminar zone and retrodiscal pad) are contiguous. The retrodiscal tissue is a soft, areolar connective tissue with large vascular spaces. The posterior attachment tissues adhere to the tympanic plate of the temporal bone posterosuperiorly and to the neck of the condyle posteroinferiorly. Anteriorly, the disk, the capsule, and the fascia of the superior head of the lateral pterygoid muscle are contiguous. The superior head of the lateral pterygoid muscle may have some fibers inserting directly into the disk anteromedially.

The articular disk of the TMJ is a hypovascular intra-articular structure that separates the condylar head from the glenoid fossa. It is firmly attached to the condyle at its lateral pole; it

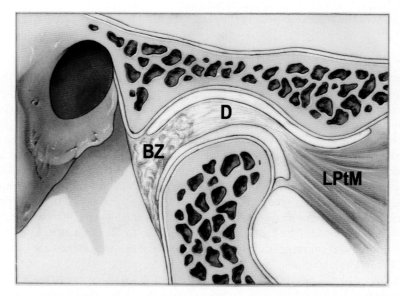

FIGURE 12.4 Sagittal section through the temporomandibular joint (TMJ). The articular disk (*D*) is *white* because of its avascularity. The bilaminar zone (*BZ*) is *red* because of its lush blood supply. The lateral pterygoid muscle (*LPtM*) may have some fibers that attach to the anterior portion of the disk.

is not directly attached to the temporal bone. The articular disk and its posterior attachment tissues merge with the capsule around their periphery. The disk and its attachments divide the joint space into separate superior and inferior spaces. In the sagittal plane, the upper joint space is contiguous with the glenoid fossa and the articular eminence. The upper joint space always extends further anteriorly than the lower joint space. The lower joint space is contiguous with the condyle and extends only slightly anterior to the condyle along the superior aspect of the superior head of the lateral pterygoid muscle. In the frontal plane, the upper joint space overlaps the lower joint space. Therefore, dissection through the lateral capsule brings one into the superior compartment.

Layers of the Temporoparietal Region

The *temporoparietal fascia* is the most superficial fascial layer beneath the subcutaneous fat (see Fig. 12.5). This fascia is the lateral extension of the galea and is continuous with the superficial musculoaponeurotic system (SMAS) layer. It is frequently called the *superficial temporal fascia* or the *suprazygomatic SMAS*. It is easy to miss this layer completely when incising the skin because it is just beneath the surface. The blood vessels of the scalp, such as the superficial temporal vessels, run along its superficial aspect close to the subcutaneous fat. On the other hand, the motor nerves, such as the temporal branch of the facial nerve, run on the deep surface of the temporoparietal fascia.

The *subgaleal fascia* in the temporoparietal region is well developed and can be dissected as a discrete fascial layer if required, but it is generally used only as a cleavage plane in the standard preauricular approach.

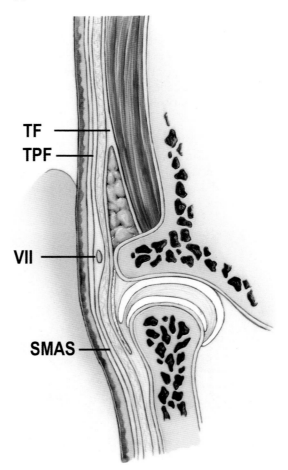

FIGURE 12.5 Coronal section of the temporomandibular joint (TMJ) region. *TF*, temporalis fascia (note that it splits inferior to this point into superficial and deep layers); *TPF*, temporoparietal fascia; *VII*, temporal branch of the facial nerve; *SMAS*, superficial musculoaponeurotic system.

The *temporalis fascia* is the fascia of the temporalis muscle. This thick fascia rises from the superior temporal line and fuses with the pericranium. The temporalis muscle rises from the deep surface of the temporal fascia and the whole of the temporal fossa. Inferiorly, at the level of the superior orbital rim, the temporal fascia splits into the superficial layer attaching to the lateral border, and the deep layer attaching to the medial border of the zygomatic arch. A small quantity of fat between the two layers is sometimes called the *superficial temporal fat pad*. A large vein frequently runs just deep to the superficial layer of temporalis fascia.

Technique

Several approaches to the TMJ have been proposed and are used clinically. The standard and most basic is the preauricular approach. Other approaches differ in the placement of the skin incision, as well as access to the joint. The dissection down to the TMJ, however, is similar in all approaches. In this chapter, the standard preauricular approach is described first. Later, the variations are presented briefly.

➤ **STEP 1.** Preparation of the Surgical Site

Preparation and draping should expose the entire ear and lateral canthus of the eye. Shaving the preauricular hair is optional. A sterile plastic drape can be used to keep the hair out of the surgical field. Cotton soaked in mineral oil or antibiotic ointment may be placed in the external auditory canal.

➤ **STEP 2.** Marking the Incision

The incision is outlined at the junction of the facial skin with the helix of the ear. A natural skin fold along the entire length of the ear can be used for incision. If none is present, posterior digital pressure applied on the preauricular skin usually creates a skin fold that can be marked (see Fig. 12.6A). The incision extends superiorly to the top of the helix and may include an anterior (hockey-stick) extension (Fig. 12.6B).

➤ **STEP 3.** Infiltration of Vasoconstrictor

The preauricular area is quite vascular. A vasoconstrictor can be injected subcutaneously in the area of the incision to decrease incisional bleeding. However, if local anesthesia is also being injected, it should not be injected deeply because it may be necessary to use a nerve stimulator on exposed facial nerve branches.

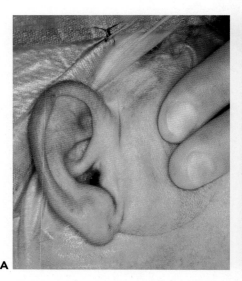 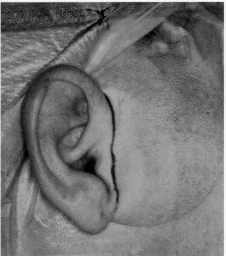

A   **B**

FIGURE 12.6 Photographs showing the method of marking skin incision. Digital pressure applied posteriorly on the skin will cause the skin to form a crease **(A)**. This crease is marked for incision **(B)**.

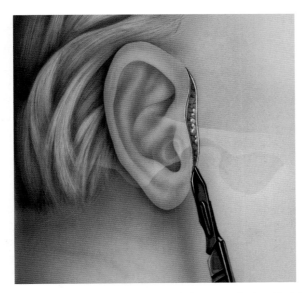

FIGURE 12.7 Illustration showing initial incision made in the preauricular skin fold.

➤ **STEP 4.** Skin Incision

The incision is made through skin and subcutaneous connective tissues (including temporoparietal fascia) to the depth of the temporalis fascia (superficial layer) (see Fig. 12.7). Any bleeding skin vessels are cauterized before proceeding with deeper dissection.

➤ **STEP 5.** Dissection to the Temporomandibular Joint Capsule

Blunt dissection with periosteal elevators and/or scissors (see Fig. 12.8A) undermines the *superior portion* of the incision (that the part above the zygomatic arch) such that a flap can be

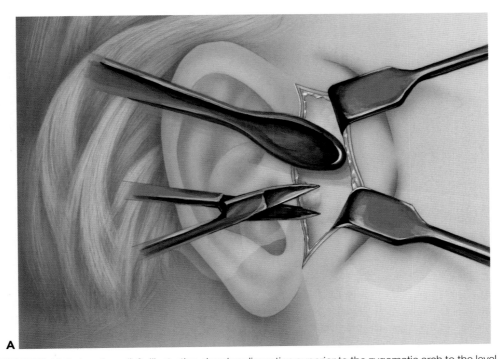

A

FIGURE 12.8 (*continued*) **A:** Illustration showing dissection superior to the zygomatic arch to the level of the superficial layer of the temporalis fascia using a periosteal elevator. The flap is dissected anteriorly at this depth. Dissection with scissors below the zygomatic arch is just anterior to (on the cartilage of) the external auditory meatus to the same depth.   (*continued*)

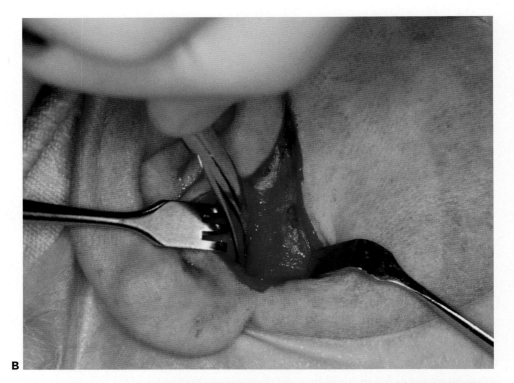

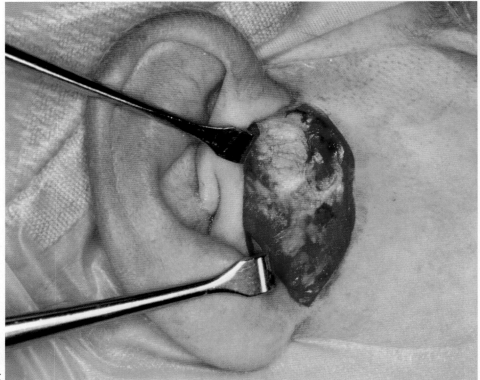

FIGURE 12.8 (*continued*) **B:** Photograph showing dissection along external auditory meatus with scissors. **C:** Photograph after dissection is complete. The superficial layer of the temporalis fascia is seen above the zygomatic arch (*white*).

retracted anteriorly for approximately 1.5 to 2 cm (Fig. 12.8B). This flap is dissected anteriorly at the level of the superficial (outer) layer of temporalis fascia. This layer is usually hypovascular. The superficial temporal vessels and auriculotemporal nerve may be retracted anteriorly in the flap. Failure to develop the flap close to the cartilaginous external auditory canal increases the risk of damage to these structures.

Below the zygomatic arch, dissection proceeds bluntly, adjacent to the external auditory cartilage. Scissor dissection proceeds along the external auditory cartilage in an avascular plane between it and the glenoid lobe of the parotid gland (Fig. 12.8B). The external auditory cartilage runs anteromedially, and the dissection is parallel to the cartilage. The depth of the dissection at this point should be similar to that above the zygomatic arch (Fig. 12.8C).

Attention is again focussed on the portion of the incision above the zygomatic arch. With the flap retracted anteriorly, an incision is made through the superficial (outer) layer of temporalis fascia, beginning at the root of the zygomatic arch just in front of the tragus, anterosuperiorly toward the upper corner of the retracted flap (see Fig. 12.9). The fat globules contained between the superficial and deep layers of the temporalis fascia are then exposed. At the root of the zygoma, the incision can be made through both the superficial layer of temporalis fascia and the periosteum of the zygomatic arch. The sharp end of a periosteal elevator is inserted in the fascial incision, deep to the superficial layer of the temporalis fascia, and swept back and forth to dissect this tissue from the underlying areolar and adipose tissues (see Fig. 12.10). The undermining proceeds inferiorly toward the zygomatic arch, where the sharp end of the periosteal elevator cleaves the attachment of the periosteum at the junction of the lateral and superior surfaces of the zygomatic arch, freeing the periosteum from its lateral surface. The periosteal elevator can then be used to continue dissecting bluntly inferiorly with a back and forth motion, taking care not to dissect medially into the TMJ capsule (Fig. 12.10). Blunt scissors can also be used to dissect inferiorly to the zygomatic arch. Once the dissection is

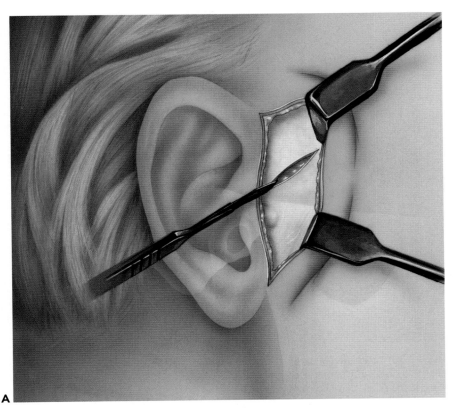

A

FIGURE 12.9 A: Illustration and **(B)** photograph showing oblique incision through the superficial layer of the temporalis fascia. Fat is visible deep to the fascia.   *(continued)*

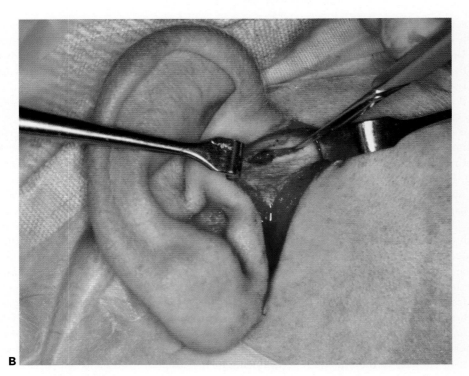

B

FIGURE 12.9 *(continued)*

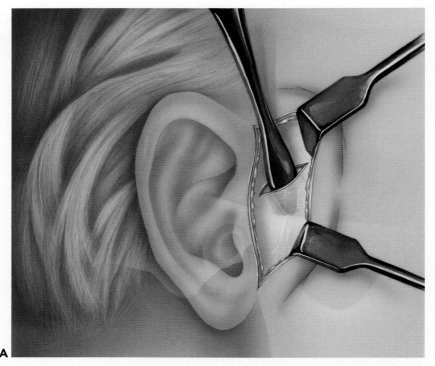

A

FIGURE 12.10 Illustration **(A)** and photograph **(B)** showing the use of a periosteal elevator inserted beneath the superficial layer of the temporalis fascia to strip the periosteum off the lateral portion of the zygomatic arch. Blunt dissection inferiorly continues below the zygomatic arch just superficial to the capsule of the temporomandibular joint. **C:** Coronal section showing the layer of dissection.

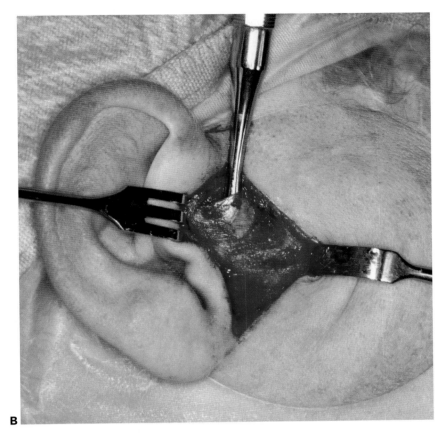

B

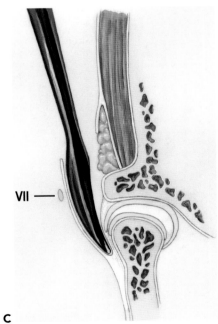

VII —

C

FIGURE 12.10 *(continued)*

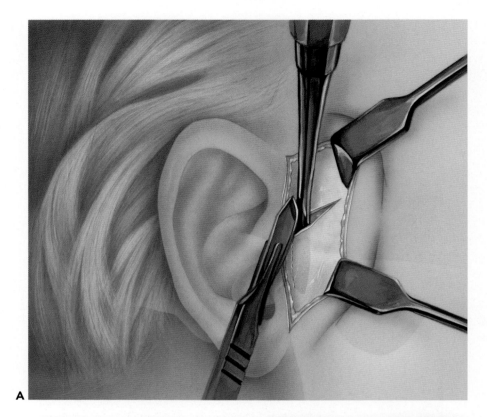

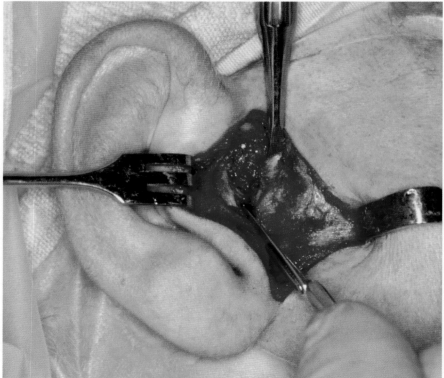

FIGURE 12.11 Illustration **(A)** and photograph **(B)** showing a vertical incision made through intervening tissues just in front of the external auditory meatus to the depth of the periosteal elevator.

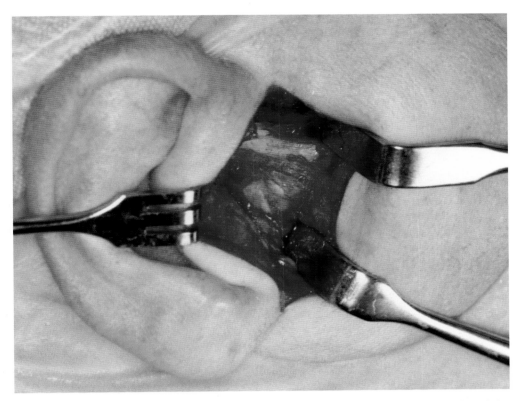

FIGURE 12.12 Photograph showing the capsule of the temporomandibular joint (TMJ) and the exposed zygomatic arch.

approximately 1 cm below the arch, the intervening tissue is sharply released posteriorly along the plane of the initial incision (see Fig. 12.11).

The entire flap is then retracted anteriorly, and blunt dissection at this depth (just superficial to the capsule of the TMJ) proceeds anteriorly until the articular eminence is exposed. The entire TMJ capsule should then be revealed (see Fig. 12.12). Because of subperiosteal dissection along the lateral surface of the zygomatic arch, the temporal branches of the facial nerve are located within the substance of the retracted flap (Fig. 12.10C). To help determine the location of the articular space, the mandible can be manipulated open and closed.

➤ STEP 6. Exposing the Interarticular Spaces

With retraction of the developed flap, the joint spaces can be entered. To facilitate the surgery, a vasoconstrictor-containing solution can be injected into the superior joint space (see Fig. 12.13). With the condyle distracted inferiorly, pointed scissors or a scalpel is used to enter the upper joint space anteriorly along the posterior slope of the eminence (see Fig. 12.14). The opening is extended anteroposteriorly by cutting along the lateral aspect of the eminence and fossa. The incision is continued inferiorly along the posterior portion of the capsule until the capsule blends with the posterior attachment of the disk. Lateral retraction of the capsule allows entrance into the superior joint space (see Fig. 12.15).

The inferior joint space is opened by making an incision in the disk along its lateral attachment to the condyle within the lateral recess of the upper joint space (see Fig. 12.16). The incision may be extended posteriorly into the posterior attachment tissues. The inferior joint space is then entered. The articular disk can be lifted superiorly or inferiorly, exposing either joint space (see Fig. 12.17).

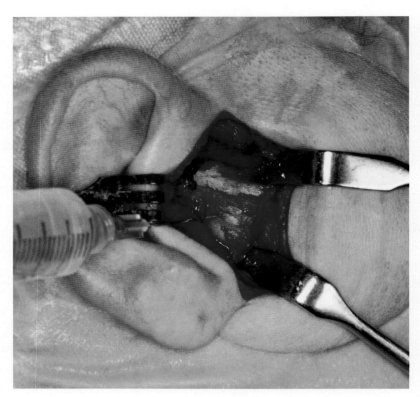

FIGURE 12.13 Photograph showing the injection of local anesthetic with epinephrine into the superior joint space.

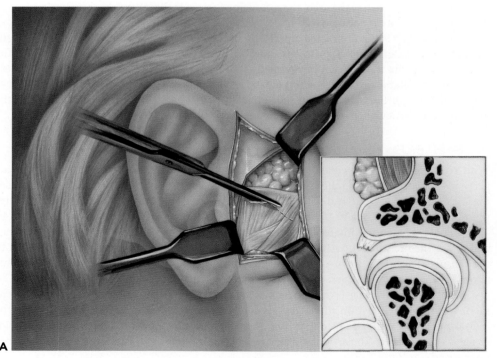

A

FIGURE 12.14 After retraction of the tissues superficial to the temporomandibular joint (TMJ) capsule, scissors **(A)** or a scalpel **(B)** is used to enter the capsule. Initial point of entry is just below the zygomatic arch; the incision will continue parallel to the contour of the temporomandibular joint (TMJ) fossa. **Inset:** Coronal section showing dissection into the superior joint space.

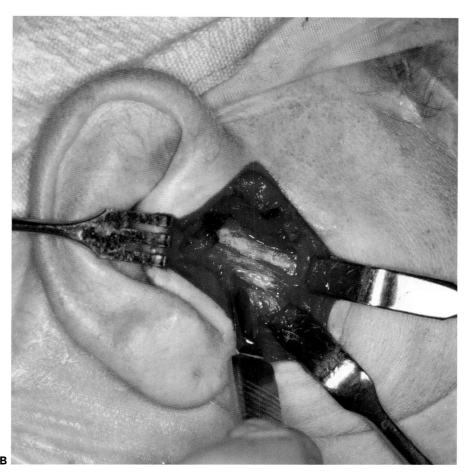

B

FIGURE 12.14 *(continued)*

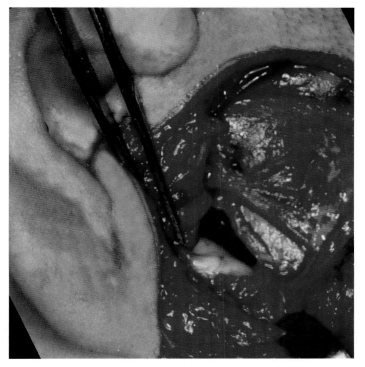

FIGURE 12.15 Photograph showing inner portion of superior joint space. The forceps is grasping the lateral portion of the articular disk (*white*).

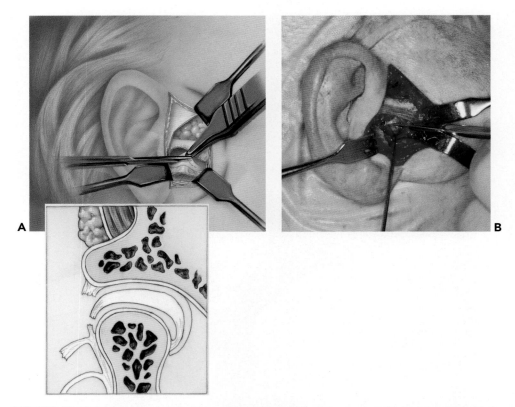

FIGURE 12.16 Incision through the lateral attachment of the temporomandibular joint disk, entering the inferior joint space. **A:** Illustration showing use of sharp scissors to incise the lateral attachment of the disk. **B:** Photograph showing a scalpel used for the same purpose. **Inset:** Coronal section showing dissection into the inferior joint space.

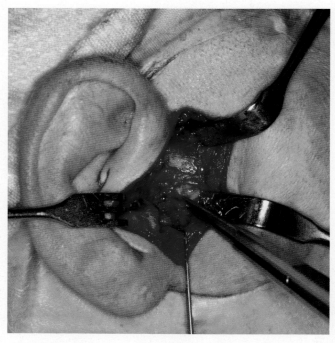

FIGURE 12.17 Photograph after the lateral attachment of the temporomandibular joint (TMJ) disk has been incised. The articular disk (forceps) can now be lifted upward to expose the condylar surface.

➤ **STEP 7.** Closure

The joint spaces are irrigated thoroughly, and any hemorrhage is controlled before closure. The inferior joint space is closed with permanent or slowly resorbing suture by suturing the disk back to its lateral condylar attachment (see Fig. 12.18). The superior joint space is closed by suturing the incised edge with the remaining capsular attachments on the temporal component of the TMJ (see Fig. 12.19). If no such attachments are left attached to bone, the capsule can be resuspended over the zygomatic arch to the temporalis fascia.

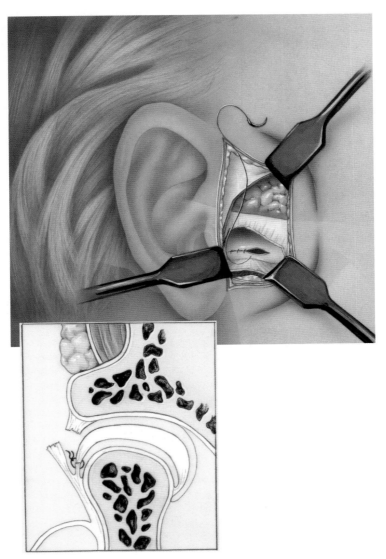

FIGURE 12.18 Closure of the inferior joint space using running suture between lateral disk attachments and the joint capsule. **Inset:** Coronal section showing suturing of articular disk.

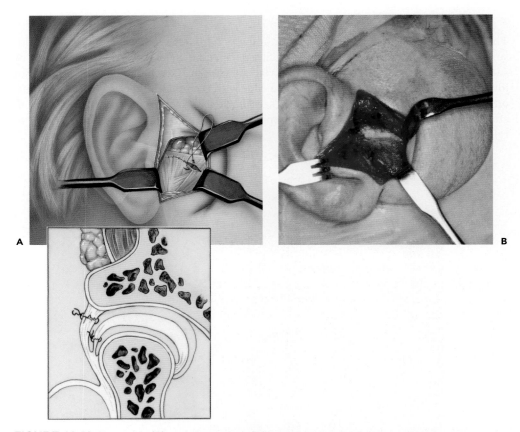

A

B

FIGURE 12.19 Illustration **(A)** and photograph **(B)** showing closure of the superior joint space using running suture between remnants of the temporomandibular joint (TMJ) capsule on the zygomatic arch and the TMJ capsule below. **Inset:** Coronal section showing suturing of articular disk and lateral capsule.

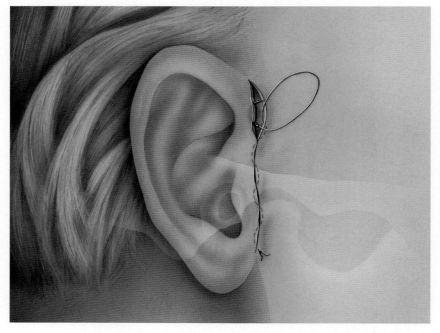

FIGURE 12.20 Closure of the preauricular skin incision with running subcuticular suture.

Subcutaneous tissues are closed with resorbable suture. No suture deeper than the subcutaneous tissues is required. The skin is then closed. A running subcuticular suture makes removal simple and allows a delay in removal if necessary (see Fig. 12.20). A pressure dressing is usually applied, taking care to bolster posterior to the ear.

Alternate Approaches

Other approaches to the TMJ have been described and used clinically. The extended temporal and coronal incisions can proceed inferiorly in the same manner as for a preauricular incision to expose the TMJ. The "extended" preauricular approach is used by some surgeons to improve the ability to retract the tissues anteriorly. The extended preauricular incision is similar to the preauricular approach, but an anterosuperior extension (hockey-stick) is made in the hair-bearing temporal skin (see Fig. 12.21). Some surgeons choose to bring the preauricular incision behind the tragus (endaural incision) to hide a portion of it (see Fig. 12.22). This choice may be especially useful in those individuals, often young patients, who do not have a well-demarcated preauricular skin fold. A retroauricular skin incision further hides the incision and helps protect the auriculotemporal nerve. This approach requires an arc-shaped incision behind the ear (see Fig. 12.23). The external auditory canal must be transected at a wide portion to prevent stenosis, and the ear is reflected anteriorly to gain access to the joint. The same deeper dissection is effective for all the approaches just described.

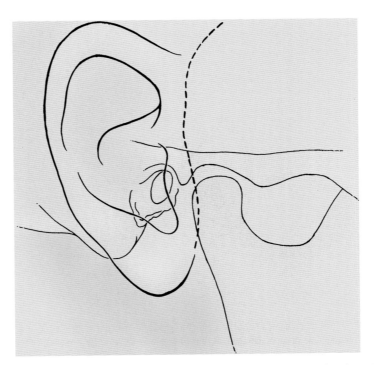

FIGURE 12.21 Preauricular incision with an oblique anterosuperior extension (hockey-stick).

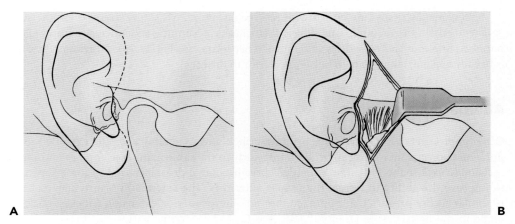

FIGURE 12.22 Preauricular incision with a retrotragal portion, hiding the scar within the ear. **A:** Incision outlined. **B:** Exposure of TMJ capsule.

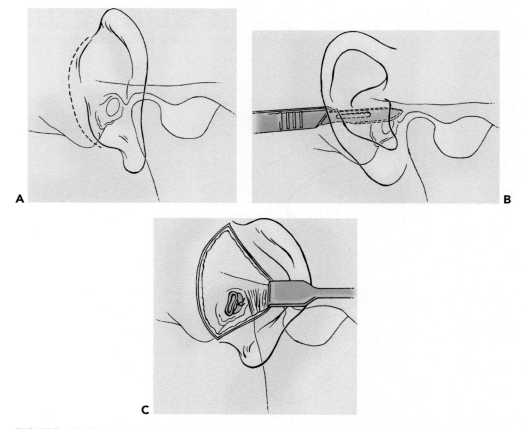

FIGURE 12.23 Retroauricular approach to the temporomandibular joint (TMJ). **A:** Initial curvilinear incision in the retroauricular crease. **B:** Transection of the external auditory meatus. **C:** Retraction of the external ear anteriorly, exposing the TMJ capsule.

REFERENCE

1. Al-Kayat A, Bramley P, A modified pre-auricular approach to the temporomandibular joint and malar arch. *Br J Oral Maxillofac Surg.* 1979;17:91.

Surgical Approaches to the Nasal Skeleton

A myriad of surgical approaches have been described to expose the nasal skeleton. Two common basic surgical approaches are described here, each with its own set of incisions and modifications. The closed or endonasal approach places all incisions within the nasal cavity so that they are inconspicuous. The open or external approach combines internal and external incisions. This section is divided into two chapters on the basis of these two approaches. Surgical anatomy is discussed in Chapter 13.

13

External (Open) Approach

The nasal skeleton is exposed during many procedures, such as rhinoplasty, septoplasty, fracture management, and reconstructive surgery. It is the only approach described in this book that involves a skeleton that is made of both bone and cartilage.

Surgical Anatomy

The nose has the form of a triangular pyramid, with its summit corresponding to the root of the nose and a base into which the two nostrils open.

External Nasal Bony Framework

The bony framework of the nose consists of the paired nasal bones, supported posteriorly by the nasal process of the frontal bone and laterally by the frontal processes of the maxilla (see Fig. 13.1). The nasal bones vary in length, constituting from one third to one half of the nasal framework. They are paired quadrilateral bones that are thick and narrow in their upper portion, becoming wider and thinner in the lower portion. The superficial surface is smooth and concave in the upper half and convex in the lower half. The inferior edge of the nasal bones is continuous with the upper lateral (triangular) cartilages, which extend underneath the nasal bones 4 to 7 mm (often called the *keystone area*).

External Nasal Cartilage Framework

The *upper lateral (triangular) cartilages* are paired structures that form the greater part of the middle one third of the lateral nasal wall (Fig. 13.1). Their medial borders fuse with the lateral expansions of the anterior border of the septal cartilage in its upper two thirds. In the lower one third, they are separated from the septum and are attached by intervening connective tissue. The upper border of the upper lateral cartilage inserts onto the deep surface of the inferior edge of the nasal bones for a few millimeters. The periosteum of the nasal bones becomes the perichondrium of the cartilage nasal skeleton at this junction. The lateral border of the upper lateral cartilage joins the piriform aperture of the maxilla. The inferior edge of the upper lateral cartilage slides under the lateral crus of the alar cartilage to which it is joined by a dense tissue, which is a prolongation of the superficial and deep perichondrial layers that include several fragments of cartilage called *sesamoids*. The attachment between the alar and upper lateral cartilages is often folded back by 2 to 3 mm and is frequently called the *scroll area* (see Fig. 13.2).

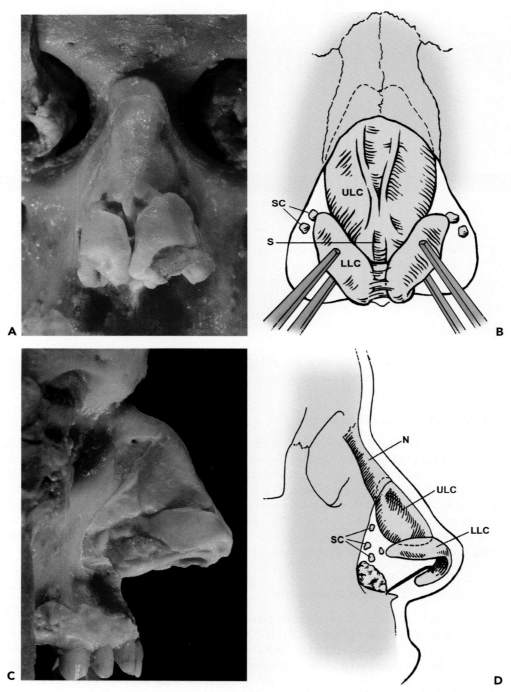

FIGURE 13.1 External skeleton of the nose. *N*, nasal bone; *ULC*, upper lateral cartilage; *SC*, sesamoid cartilages; *S*, cartilaginous septum; *LLC*, lower lateral cartilage.

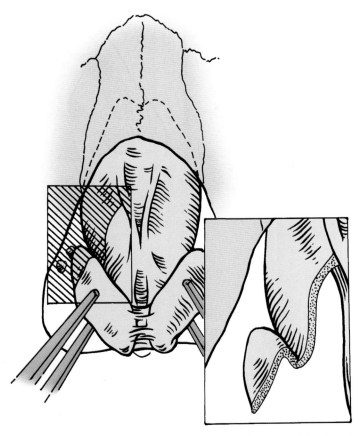

FIGURE 13.2 Scroll area where upper and lower lateral cartilages are joined by fibrocartilaginous tissue.

The *alar (lower lateral) cartilages* are paired structures that have medial and lateral crura. The two medial crura come together at the midline and take part in forming the columella (see Fig. 13.3). The posteroinferior edges of the medial crura diverge (foot plates) and attach to the septal cartilage by fibrous tissue. The lateral crura are quadrangular and usually convex. They contribute little to the shape or structure of the ala, which is primarily a fibrofatty structure. The length of the lateral crura varies considerably from one individual to another, but their outline is usually visible through the overlying skin. The lateral border of the lateral crura extends toward the piriform aperture but does not reach it being connected by intervening connective tissue and sesamoid cartilage islands (Figs. 13.1 and 13.2). The height of the lateral crura also varies widely, with a mean of approximately 11 mm. The superior edge of the lateral crura overlies the inferior edge of the upper lateral cartilage. The inferior border of the lateral crus does not follow the alar rim and is closer to the rim medially, where it may be 5 to 6 mm posterior. Laterally, the inferior edge of the lateral crus may be 12 to 14 mm superior to the alar rim (Fig. 13.1). Therefore, the inferior border of the lateral crus extends superiorly as it extends laterally. This relation is readily visible through the skin or by performing an endonasal examination with retraction of the alar rim. The junction of the medial and lateral crus can be abrupt, forming an acute angle, or genu. In some instances, a flat area is noted between them, giving rise to the term *middle crus*. The alar cartilages are attached by interdomal ligamentous attachments, which extend over the top of the cartilaginous septal angle, contributing to tip support (Fig. 13.3).

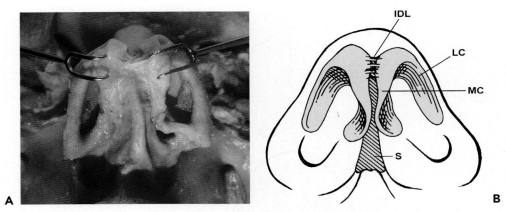

FIGURE 13.3 Base of the nose. *IDL*, interdomal ligaments; *LC*, lateral crus of the lower lateral cartilage; *MC*, medial crus of the lower lateral cartilage; *S*, septum.

The Nasal Septum

The septum of the nose is made of six structures; the septal crest of the maxilla, the perpendicular plate of the palatine bone, the perpendicular plate of the ethmoid bone, the vomer, the cartilaginous septum (quadrangular cartilage), and the membranous septum (see Fig. 13.4). The *cartilaginous septum (quadrangular cartilage)* is an anterior extension of the bony septum; it has a roughly quadrangular shape. The anterosuperior border contributes to the nasal bridge. In its upper one third, this border is located under the deep surface of the nasal bones. In its middle one third, it is in close relation to the upper lateral cartilages; the anterior septal border enlarges to form two lateral expansions that articulate with the medial borders of the upper lateral cartilages through a dense fibrous articulation. The anterior border of the septum is wide superiorly and narrows as it proceeds downward. The *anterior septal angle* is at the junction of the dorsal and caudal septa. In its lower one third, the septal cartilage is separated from the upper lateral cartilages and is clearly behind the alar cartilages. An anteroinferior border, extending obliquely posterior, forms a rounded angle with the anterior nasal spine to which it is firmly bound by the perichondrial and periosteal tissues that extend around it at this level to form a tight but somewhat mobile articulation. A posterosuperior border is joined to the perpendicular plate of the ethmoid by a tight attachment. The posteroinferior border extends obliquely from posterior to anterior. This flared border narrows posteriorly and has a caudal prolongation that extends between the ethmoid and the vomer. Anteriorly, the inferior border expands to install itself on the incisive crest that sometimes becomes a groove to hold this border.

Nasal Soft Tissues

The soft tissues covering the nose consist of skin, a complex musculoaponeurotic sheath, and the periosteum/perichondrium. The arteries and veins of the nose are in the soft tissues. Therefore, the plane of dissection in nasal surgeries should be close to the osteo-cartilaginous framework to avoid injuring these muscles and vessels. The nasal soft tissues are important in understanding the effect of certain surgical procedures on nasal function and esthetics. However, for the purpose of exposure of the nasal skeleton, these factors are less important because the dissection is made in the subperiosteal/subperichondrial plane.

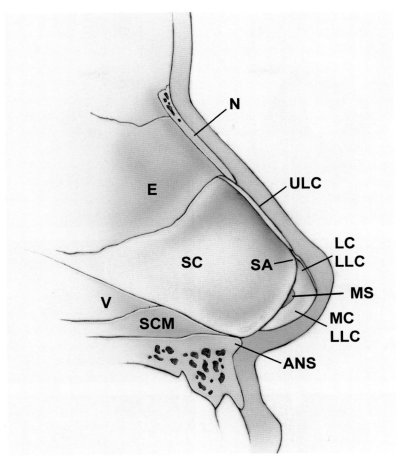

FIGURE 13.4 Components of the nasal septum. *N*, nasal bone; *ULC*, cut edge of the upper lateral cartilage; *E*, ethmoid; *SC*, septal cartilage; *SA*, septal angle; *V*, vomer; *SCM*, septal crest of the maxilla; *LC, LLC*, cut edge of the lateral crus, lower lateral cartilage; *MS*, membranous septum; *MC, LLC*, medial crus, lower lateral cartilage; *ANS*, anterior nasal spine.

Technique

The external approach to the nasal skeleton involves only one external incision placed across the columella. This approach consists of bilateral marginal incisions connected by a transcolumellar incision. The soft tissue is elevated off the cartilages and nasal bones, exposing the entire tip and dorsum.

➤ **STEP 1.** Vasoconstriction and Preparation

The vibrissae within the vestibules are shaved with a no. 15 scalpel or scissors and the nasal cavity is cleaned with a povidone–iodine solution. A combination of intranasal packs and vasoconstrictor injections can help with hemostasis during the surgery. Nasal packing with a vasoconstrictor (4% cocaine, 0.05% oxymetazoline, etc.) is placed along the length of the nasal floor, against the turbinates and under the osteocartilaginous roof. Local infiltration of a vasoconstrictor induces hemostasis and assists dissection by separating tissue planes. The infiltration is carried out between the skin and the osteocartilaginous skeleton, trying to deform the overlying skin as little as possible, and submucosally (see Fig. 13.5). After infiltration, gentle external pressure applied over the nose for 1 to 2 minutes helps spread the vasoconstrictor homogeneously, thereby reducing the external deformity. The external structures are then prepared in a standard manner.

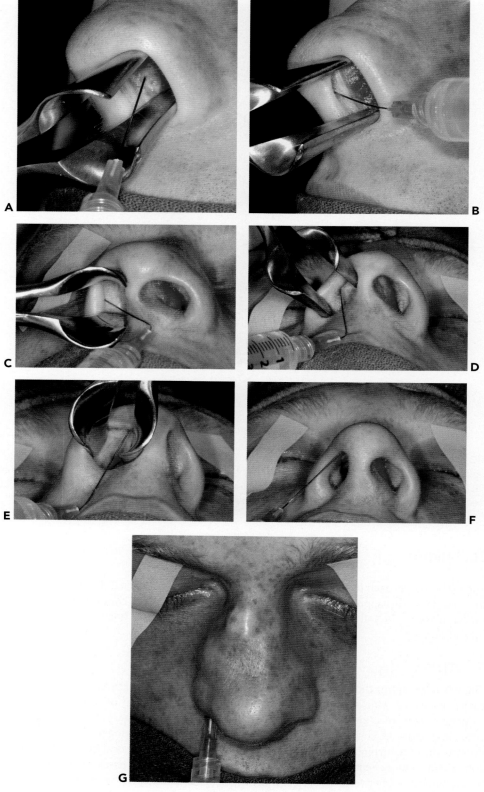

FIGURE 13.5 Photographs showing the injection of a vasoconstrictor to assist in hemostasis and develop a plane of dissection. **(A)** Submucosal injection of the nasal septum; **(B)**, injection of the membranous septum and along the medial crus of the lower lateral cartilage; **(C–E)**, injection along the location of the marginal incision; **(F)**, injection of the nasal dome; **(G)**, injection just superficial to the upper lateral cartilages and the nasal bones.

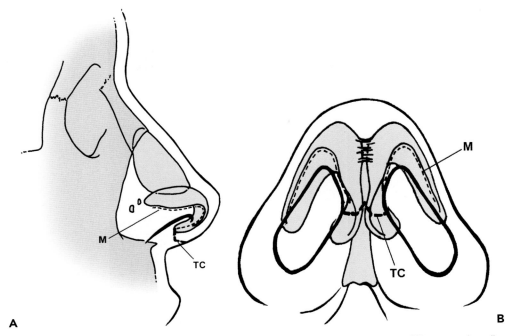

FIGURE 13.6 A and **B:** Incisions for an external approach. *M,* marginal incision; *TC,* transcolumellar incision. Note how the marginal incision follows the caudal border of the lower lateral cartilage.

➤ STEP 2. Marginal and Transcolumellar Incisions

The incisions for the open approach should be marked with a fine-tipped marking pen. The *marginal incision* for exposure of the dome and lateral crus should follow the free caudal margin of the lower lateral cartilage and not the margin of the nostril (see Fig. 13.6). Incisions should not be placed into the soft triangle, which is the portion of the nostril caudal to the alar cartilage. The soft triangle is formed by two juxtaposed layers of skin, unsupported by cartilage, with only loose areolar tissue between them, and any incision made may result in disfiguring postoperative notching. This possible result is why the rim incision, which requires dissection through the soft triangle, is best avoided.

The nostril rim is retracted with a double skin hook and everted by placing the middle finger externally over the alar cartilage. The caudal edge of the alar cartilage is identified through the vestibular skin (see Fig. 13.7A). The positioning of the inferior border of the lateral crus in relation to the alar rim has been discussed earlier. The back of the scalpel handle can be used to palpate the caudal border of the alar cartilage.

The marginal incision continues medially to the apex and along the caudal rim of the medial crus, approximately 1 mm behind the rim of the columella, stopping at the columella–lobule junction (Fig. 13.7B). The incision should stop medially at the narrowest point of the columella between the columella–lobule junction and the flare of the feet of the medial crura. A *transcolumellar* incision is marked as either a stair-step (Fig. 13.7C) or an inverted-V incision (Fig. 13.7D) in the skin across the columella, connecting to the ends of the marginal incision.

Once marked, the incisions can be made. Personal preference dictates whether the transcolumellar incision or the marginal incision is to be made first. If the marginal incision is made first, it is usually made from lateral to medially, following the contour of the alar cartilage through the vestibular skin to the level of the cartilage (see Fig. 13.8). Care must be taken not to incise too deeply in the middle and lateral crus areas, where the cartilage is very superficial. Once the marginal incision has been completed, the transcolumellar incision is made with a no. 11 blade (see Fig. 13.9). The medial crura are superficial in the columella. Therefore, skin incision across the columella should be performed carefully, or the cartilage will be inadvertently severed.

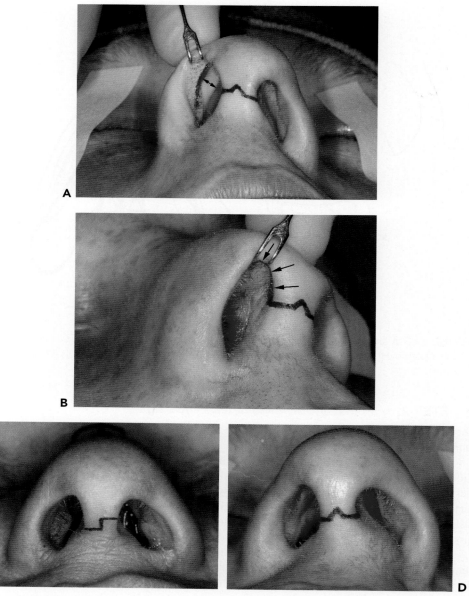

FIGURE 13.7 Photograph showing the position of the marginal incision and transcolumellar incisions. **A:** Marginal incision marked with pen. Note that it follows the caudal border of the lower lateral cartilage. The *arrow* shows the height of the lateral crus of the lower lateral cartilage. The marginal incision continues medially and anteriorly before turning inferiorly (**B**, *arrows*). The transcolumellar incision can be made as a stair-step **(C)** or an inverted-V **(D)**.

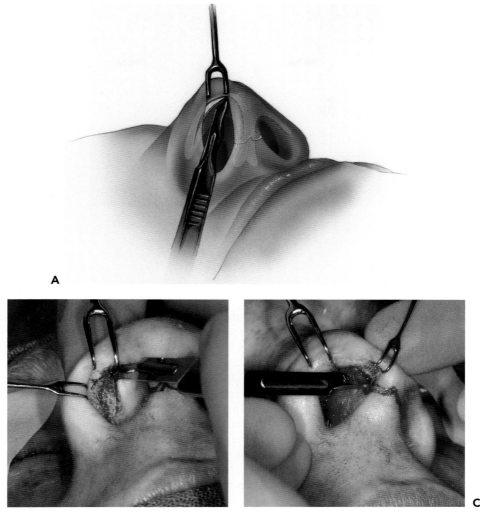

FIGURE 13.8 Marginal incision. **A:** Illustration demonstrating the marginal incision being made. Note that the lower lateral cartilage is visible through the incision. **B:** Photograph showing marginal incision being made, beginning laterally and extending medially. Note how the skin hook retracts the alar rim superiorly while a finger presses the alar cartilage downward and outward. **C:** The marginal incision continues along the anterior border of the middle and medial crus of the lower lateral cartilage, just behind the columella.

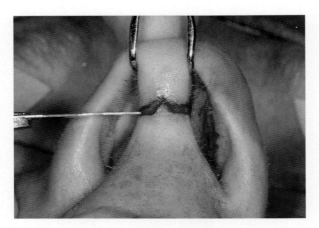

FIGURE 13.9 Photograph showing transcolumellar incision being made with a no. 11 scalpel.

➤ **STEP 3.** External Skeletonization of the Nose

A skin hook or fine forceps is used to lift the cut edge of the columellar skin gently to allow subperichondrial dissection of the medial crura with scissors. The overlying soft tissues are thin and will tear readily if dissection is not made in the subperichondrial plane. Dissection across the anterior portion of the medial crura frees the columellar skin (see Fig. 13.10). Brisk bleeding is often encountered in this area because of the common presence of blood vessels, which run vertically along the columella (see Fig. 13.11).

A double skin hook is then used to evert the rim of the nostril to insert pointed scissors into the marginal incision (see Fig. 13.12A). The tips of the scissors should contact the caudal edge of the lateral crus of the lower lateral cartilage and, with a spreading motion, free the entire caudal edge of adherent tissue. The tips of the scissors are then inserted superficial to the lateral crus in the subperichondrial plane and, with a spreading motion, this surface is freed from the overlying tissues (Fig. 13.12B).

At the junction of the lateral and medial crura, the dissection of the soft tissues from the skeleton is especially difficult, partly because they adhere to the interdomal ligaments (Fig. 13.12C). This area is also the point of acuteness between the medial and lateral crura, so trying to stay within the subperichondrial plane may be difficult. Once the dissection has been performed both laterally and medially, the last area to be dissected is the area of acuteness between the lateral and medial crus. Scissors can be passed from one pocket to the other, providing access to this area that is difficult to approach (Fig. 13.12D).

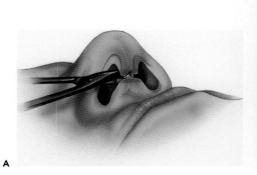
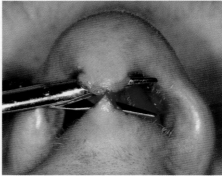

A **B**

FIGURE 13.10 Illustration **(A)** and photograph **(B)** showing the use of scissors to dissect the columellar skin off the medial cruse in the subperichondrial plane.

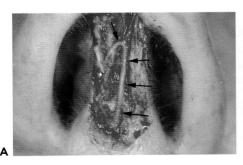
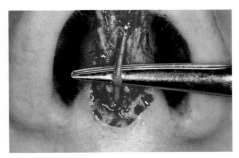

FIGURE 13.11 A and **B:** Photographs showing large columellar vein.

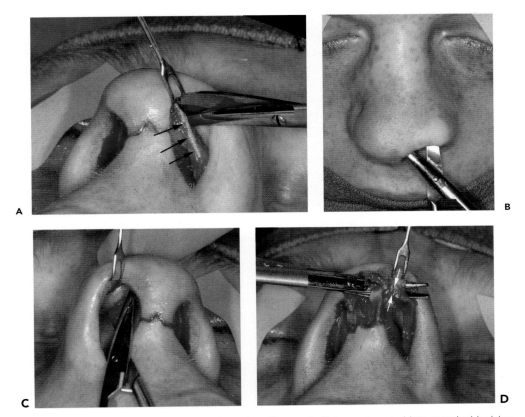

FIGURE 13.12 Dissection of the lower lateral cartilages. **A:** Scissors inserted into marginal incision just superficial to the alar cartilage (subperichondrial plane). Note the caudal edge of the alar cartilage (*arrows*). **B:** Scissor dissection superficial to the alar cartilage can be continued to the opposite side. **C:** Scissor dissection medially over the top of the alar cartilage. **D:** Scissors placed superficially to alar cartilage, showing the last area where dissection must proceed (*arrows*) to completely free the skin of the nose from the alar cartilage.

A skin hook is used to elevate the skin edges and scissors are used to dissect the remaining connections between the skin and the alar cartilages (see Fig. 13.13A). If the dissection is not in the subperichondrial plane (Fig. 13.13B), any adherent tissue remaining on the superficial surface of the lower lateral cartilage can be removed with pickups and scissor dissection. The tips of the scissors are inserted against the cartilages and with a spreading and snipping motion, the adherent tissues are freed (Fig. 13.13C and D). Subperichondrial scissor dissection proceeds superiorly and laterally toward the piriform aperture to provide as much exposure as required (Fig. 13.13E).

Once the skin and subcutaneous tissues are freed from the medial and lateral crura, the loose soft tissue overlying the anterior septal angle is incised and a similar avascular plane is identified over the lower dorsum. Downward traction with a hook on the underside of the alar cartilages facilitates this dissection. Subperichondrial dissection of the upper lateral cartilages is accomplished simply with scissors, in a spreading motion (see Fig. 13.14). On reaching the caudal margin of the nasal bones, the periosteum is incised and elevated in continuity with the overlying skin and soft tissue. The nasal bones are exposed with subperiosteal dissection using elevators until the desired areas are exposed (see Fig. 13.15).

➤ **STEP 4.** Exposing the Septum

The septum is approached by dissecting between the medial and intermediate (middle) crura with pointed scissors, through the interdomal ligament and membranous septum, exposing the caudal portion of the septal cartilage (see Fig. 13.16A and C). An incision is made along the caudal edge of the cartilaginous septum, and the mucoperichondrium is elevated off the septum (Fig. 13.16D and E). Dissection on one side of the septum should begin with a sharp instrument, such as the back of a scalpel blade or a Cottle elevator (Fig. 13.16F and G). It is difficult to establish a subperichondrial plane but is imperative to do so. Once the elevator is subperichondrial, dissection within this plane is easy. To provide more access, the upper lateral cartilage(s) can be separated from the septal cartilage. A simple method to perform the separation is by using the sharp edge of the Cottle elevator, which can readily incise through the cartilage (Fig. 13.16H). A Freer elevator can then be used to strip the entire nasal septum in a subperichondrial/subperiosteal plane (Fig. 13.16I). The difference in *feel* between cartilaginous and bony components of the nasal septum can be easily noted.

To expose the nasal septum bilaterally, dissection of the mucoperichondrium is performed on each side, to release the upper lateral cartilage from the septal cartilage. Dissection of the anterior nasal spine is also easy, through a subperichondrial dissection inferiorly and anteriorly. A nasal speculum can then be inserted, completely isolating the septum (Fig. 13.16J).

➤ **STEP 5.** Closure and Splints

The transcolumellar incision is meticulously repaired with 6-0 nylon or polypropylene suture (see Fig. 13.17). The marginal incisions are closed with 5-0 chromic catgut sutures. The sutures are placed laterally and medially, working toward the dome area. Care is needed to ensure that the cartilage is not included in the suture because it can result in the distortion of the cartilage. Any suture that distorts the nasal tip should be removed and replaced.

If the septal mucosa was detached, placement of intranasal splints or packs will maintain mucosal approximation and help prevent hematoma formation during the healing process (see Fig. 13.18). Alternatively, trans-septal quilting sutures are useful in readapting the mucosa.

An external nasal dressing may be applied to readapt the tissues to the underlying skeleton. After wiping a thin coating of tincture of benzoin or other skin preparation solution over the skin of the nose and adjoining area (see Fig. 13.19A), paper tape is applied in overlapping layers from the root to the supratip area (Fig. 13.19B and C). A strip of tape is placed to form a sling for tip support. A thermoplastic material is cut in the form of a rhombus to cover the external nasal skeleton (Fig. 13.19D). It is softened in warm water and applied to the nose, using gentle digital pressure to maintain the desired form until it is set (Fig. 13.19E and F).

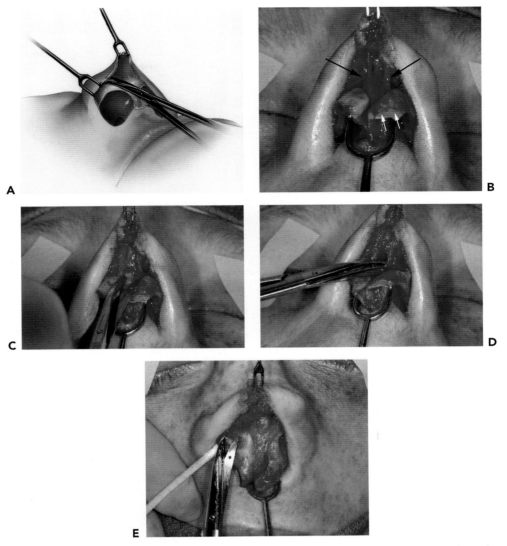

FIGURE 13.13 Continued dissection of the alar cartilages. **A:** Illustration showing scissor dissection of the nasal skin from the alar cartilages. **B:** Photograph showing initial elevation of the skin. Note that a subperichondrial dissection was performed on the patient's right alar cartilage and a supraperichondrial dissection has been performed on the patient's left (*white arrows*). Also note the connections between the septal cartilage and scroll area with the overlying skin (*black arrows*). Scissors are used to spread the remaining connections between the skin and cartilages **(C)** and then sever them **(D)**. **E:** Subperichondrial dissection laterally toward piriform aperture.

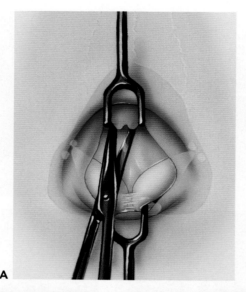

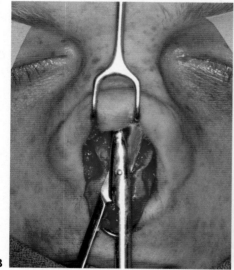

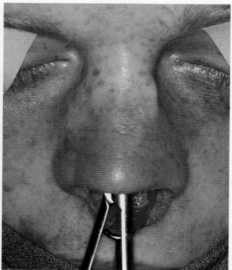

FIGURE 13.14 (A) Illustration and **(B)**, photograph showing dissection of the nasal dorsum. Double-ball hook elevates the skin of the nose, double skin hook inserted in the undersurface of alar cartilages, retracting them inferiorly, while scissors are used to dissect dorsum in the subperichondrial plane. **C:** Scissors used to dissect in the subperiosteal plane over the nasal bones.

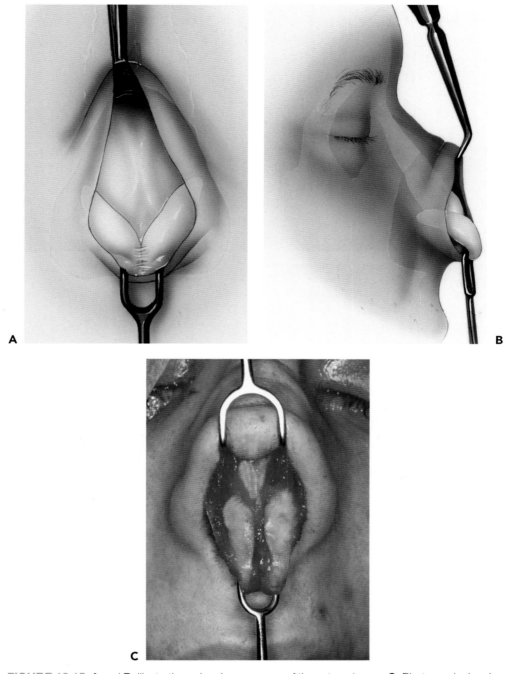

FIGURE 13.15 A and **B:** Illustrations showing exposure of the external nose. **C:** Photograph showing the same.

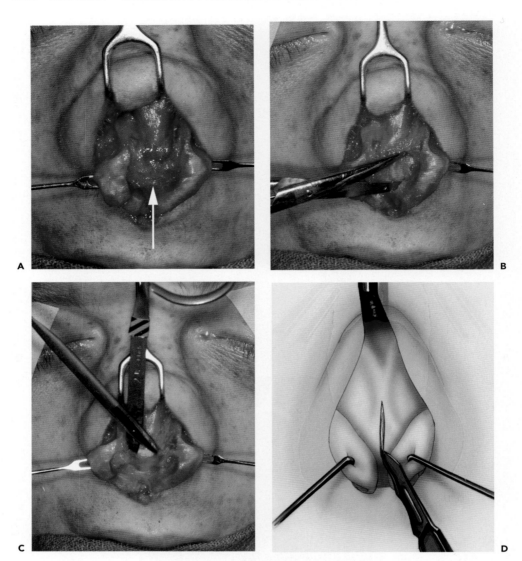

FIGURE 13.16 Exposure of the nasal septum. **A:** Double skin hooks used to separate the lower lateral cartilages. Note the interdomal ligaments (*arrow*). **B:** Scissors used to dissect through the interdomal ligaments, allowing separation of the lower lateral cartilages. **C:** Scissors used to dissect to the nasal septum. **D:** Illustration showing incision on the septal cartilage after interdomal ligaments have been removed and the membranous septum has been dissected.

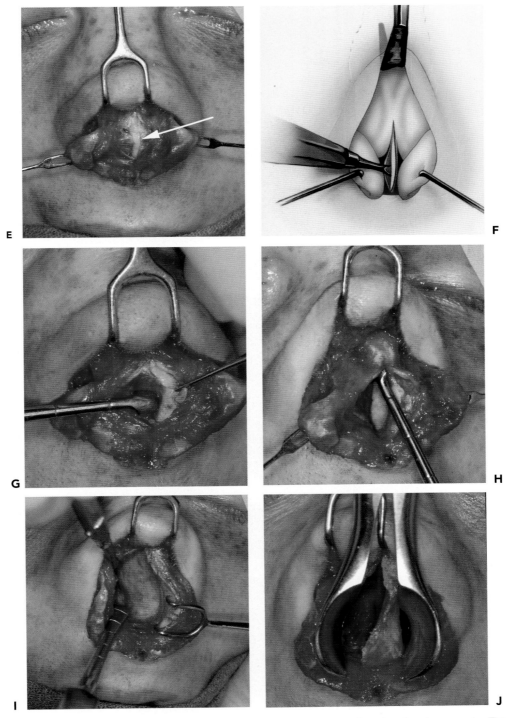

FIGURE 13.16 (*continued*) **E:** Appearance after initial incision to nasal septum has been made. The *arrow* indicates the anterior septal angle. **F:** Illustration showing the use of a sharp periosteal elevator to dissect along one side of nasal septum in subperichondrial plane. **G:** Cottle elevator used to perform subchondral dissection of nasal septal mucosa. Note skin hook providing stabilization of the septum during dissection. **H:** Cottle elevator within subchondral plane used to incise through the connection between upper lateral and septal cartilages. Note the skin hooks used to separate the lower lateral cartilages, providing access to the septum. **I:** Right side of a very deviated nasal septum has been completely exposed in a subperichondrial/subperiosteal plane. **J:** Appearance of deviated nasal septum after bilateral submucosal dissection. Note how the entire septum can be exposed using this technique.

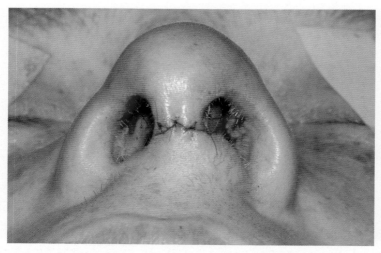

FIGURE 13.17 Closure of the transcolumellar incision.

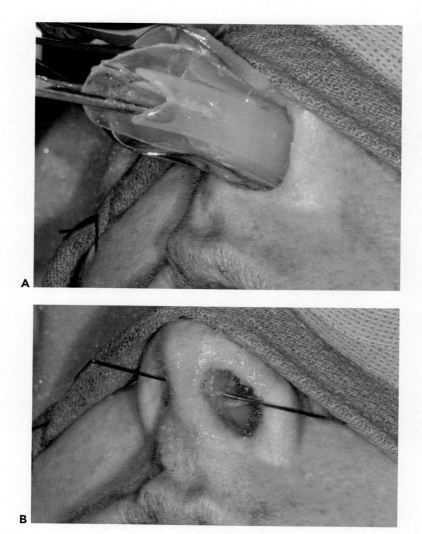

FIGURE 13.18 **A:** Insertion of silicone splint lubricated with antibiotic ointment into the nares. Note that a nasal speculum is used to create a channel for simple insertion. **B:** Bilateral silicone splints have been placed. A silk suture on a straight needle is passed through one splint, the membranous septum, and the other splint. The suture is then passed back in the opposite direction and tied.

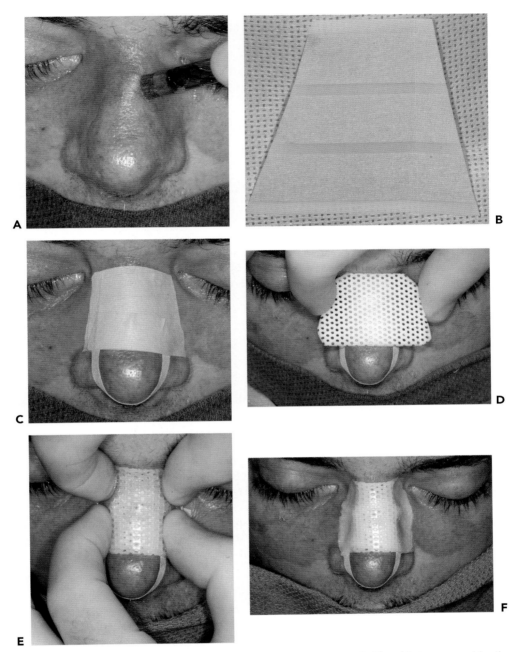

FIGURE 13.19 Application of thermoplastic splint to external nose. **A:** The skin is prepared by the application of a "sticky" material such as benzoin. **B:** Paper tape is cut into elongated rhombus and applied to the nasal skin **(C)**. **D:** Thermoplastic material cut to proper size. **E:** Softened thermoplastic dressing being adapted to the nose. **F:** Appearance after the dressing is set.

14 Endonasal Approach

Several endonasal approaches and incisions to expose the nasal skeleton have been described. The technique for modification of the alar cartilages is the major variable in the different approaches. The endonasal approach described in this chapter is the "delivery approach" for exposing the lower lateral cartilages.

Technique

➤ STEP 1. Vasoconstriction and Preparation

The vibrissae within the vestibules are shaved with a no. 15 scalpel or scissors, and the nasal cavity is cleaned with povidone–iodine solution. A combination of intranasal packs and vasoconstrictor injections helps hemostasis during the surgery. Nasal packing with a vasoconstrictor (4% cocaine, 0.05% oxymetazoline, etc.) is placed along the length of the nasal floor, against the turbinates and under the osteocartilaginous roof. Local infiltration of a vasoconstrictor provides hemostasis and assists dissection by separating tissue planes. The infiltration is carried out between the skin and the osteocartilaginous skeleton, trying to deform the overlying skin as little as possible, and submucosally. After infiltration, gentle external pressure applied over the nose for 1 to 2 minutes helps spread the vasoconstrictor homogeneously, thereby reducing external deformity. The external structures are then prepared in the standard manner.

➤ STEP 2. Cartilage Delivery Technique for Lower Lateral Cartilage Exposure

The alar cartilage delivery approach involves a marginal incision and an intercartilaginous incision connected to a partial or complete transfixion incision (see Fig. 14.1). The entire nasal skeleton can be exposed through these incisions, which are placed entirely within the nasal cavity.

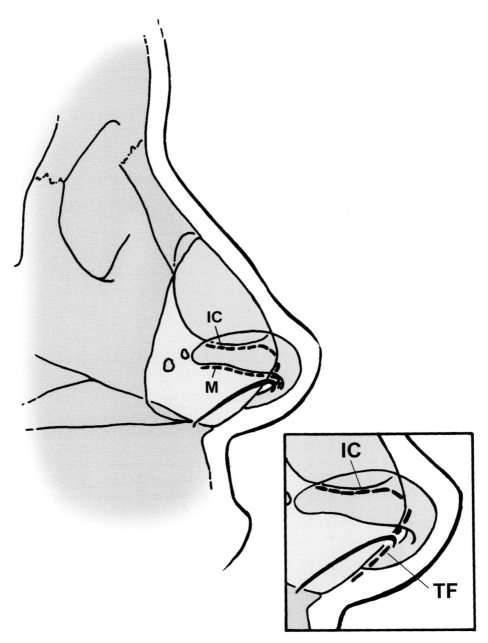

FIGURE 14.1 Incisions for the alar cartilage delivery approach. *IC*, intercartilaginous incision; *M*, marginal incision; *TF*, transfixion incision. Note how the transfixion incision follows the caudal border of the septal cartilage (***inset***).

A *marginal incision* for exposure of the dome and lateral crus should follow the free caudal margin of the lower lateral cartilage and not the margin of the nostril (see Figs. 14.1 and 14.2; see also Figs. 13.5 to 13.7). Incisions should not be placed into the soft triangle—the portion of the nostril that is caudal to the alar cartilage. The soft triangle is formed by two juxtaposed layers of skin, unsupported by cartilage, with only loose areolar tissue between. Incisions in the soft triangle may result in disfiguring postoperative notching. This possible result is why the rim incision, which requires dissection through the soft triangle, is to be avoided.

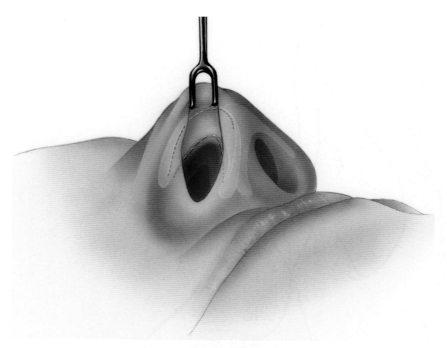

FIGURE 14.2 Retraction of the ala reveals positioning of the marginal, intercartilaginous, and transfixion incisions.

The nostril rim is retracted with a double skin hook and everted by placing the middle finger externally over the alar cartilage (Fig. 14.2). The caudal edge of the alar cartilage is identified through the vestibular skin. As described in Chapter 13, the inferior border of the lateral crus does not follow the alar rim, and is closer to the rim medially, where it may be 5 to 6 mm posterior to the alar rim. Laterally, the inferior edge of the lateral crus may be 12 to 14 mm superior to the alar rim. The inferior border of the lateral crus extends superiorly as it extends laterally (see Fig. 14.3). The back of the scalpel handle can be used to palpate the caudal border of the alar cartilage. An incision through the vestibular skin along the contour of

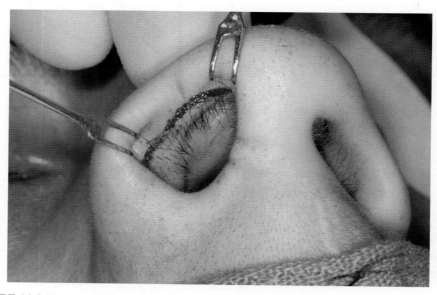

FIGURE 14.3 Photograph showing location of the marginal incision.

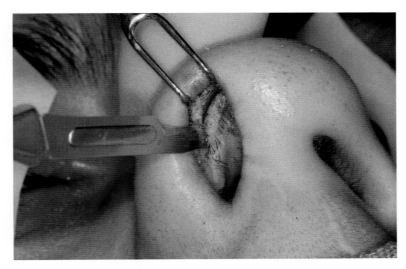

FIGURE 14.4 Photograph showing marginal incision being made. Note the skin hook retracting the alar rim superiorly while a finger placed outside the nose presses downward, facilitating the access.

the alar cartilage is made to the depth of the cartilage (see Fig. 14.4). It begins laterally beyond the point where the caudal rim of the lateral crus diverges from the alar rim to turn cephalad, follows the rim medially to the apex and continues along the caudal rim of the medial crus, approximately 1 mm behind the rim of the columella, stopping at the columella–lobule junction. If required, it can be extended further inferiorly along the medial crus and more laterally along the lateral crus to facilitate delivery of the cartilage.

The *intercartilaginous incision* (limen vestibuli incision) divides the junction of the upper and lower lateral cartilages (Figs. 14.1 and 14.2). The incision traverses the aponeurotic-like fibroareolar tissue that maintains the attachment between them (scroll area). The ala is retracted using a double skin hook and the inferior edge of the alar cartilage is identified. The skin hook elevates the alar cartilages, leaving the inferior edge of the upper lateral cartilage protruding into the vestibule, covered only by the nasal mucosa (see Fig. 14.5A). An incision is made along the inferior border of the upper lateral cartilage, beginning at the lateral end of the limen vestibuli and extending medially approximately 2 mm caudal and parallel to the limen (see Fig. 14.6A and B). It is important to make the incision 2 to 3 mm caudal to the limen vestibuli to avoid unnecessary scarring at the nasal valve area. The incision is then

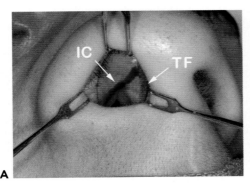
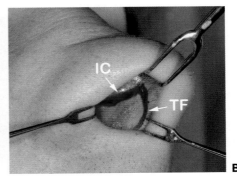

FIGURE 14.5 Frontal photograph **(A)**, and lateral photograph **(B)** showing location of intercartilaginous (*IC*) and transfixion incisions (*TF*).

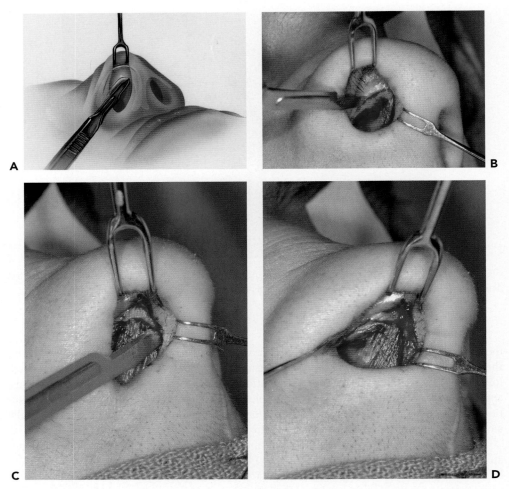

FIGURE 14.6 Illustration **(A)** and photograph **(B)**, showing intercartilaginous incision being performed. Note that the marginal incision has already been completed, exposing the lower lateral cartilage. **C:** Photograph showing hemitransfixion incision being made. **D:** Photograph after both intercartilaginous and transfixion incisions have been made.

curved into the membranous septum anterior to the valve area, where it meets the transfixion incision (Figs. 14.1, 14.2 and 14.6C). The length of the incision, which should always extend to the midline, varies with the extent of dorsum exposure necessary and alar cartilage to be freed during tip surgery.

For the cartilage delivery approach to the lower lateral cartilages, a *transfixion incision* is made at the caudal end of the septal cartilage, connecting it to the intercartilaginous incision (Figs. 14.1, 14.2 and 14.5). Transfixion is a technique in which the soft tissues overlying the dorsum and columella are separated from the septum. A hemitransfixion incision is made at the same location, but only on one side, leaving the membranous septum intact on the opposite side. The incision may extend posteriorly only to the point where it is anterior to the attachments of the posterior edges of the medial crura to the septal cartilage and its lining (partial transfixion), or it may continue posteriorly to sever the columella and lip from the septal cartilage and anterior nasal spine (complete transfixion). The transfixion incision allows complete exposure of the septum and easy delivery of the alar cartilages.

An incision is made along the caudal border of the septal cartilage, from the medial end of the intercartilaginous incision toward the anterior nasal spine (or vice versa) (Figs. 14.1 and 14.6). The length of the incision depends on whether the procedures on the anterior nasal spine and base of the septal cartilage are required. The incision is preferably placed against the caudal border of the septal cartilage, leaving the membranous septum attached to the columella. If a complete transfixion incision is necessary, it is made from one side through to the other with a scalpel and divides the membranous septum from the caudal border of the septum on both sides.

It is important to extend the transfixion incision around the septal angle to release the alar cartilages from their septal attachments when complete exposure by a marginal incision is required in the delivery approach (Fig. 14.6). To bring the dome and medial crura into view, they must not be restrained by their septal attachment.

Pointed scissors inserted into the marginal incision free the soft tissue over the alar cartilages by subperichondrial dissection (spreading motion) (see Fig. 14.7A). Elevation

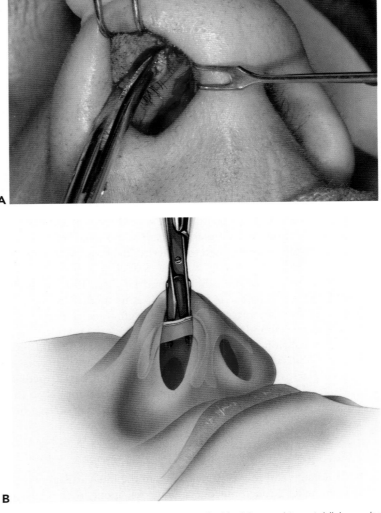

FIGURE 14.7 **A:** Scissors are inserted into the marginal incision and to establish a subperichondrial plane. **B:** Scissor dissection of the lower lateral cartilage is complete.

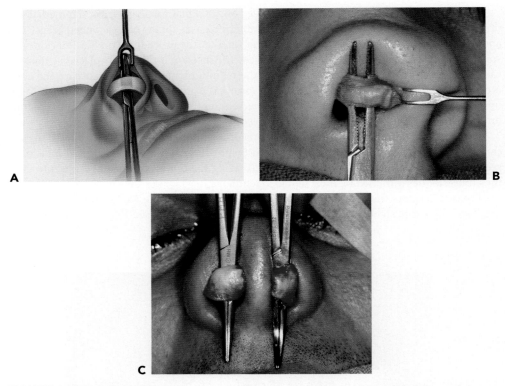

FIGURE 14.8 Illustration **(A)** and photographs **(B:** unilateral; **C:** bilateral) showing delivery of alar cartilage(s).

is carried laterally to the point of attachment of the lateral crura to the soft tissue in the region of the sesamoid cartilages. The subperichondrial dissection can be carried across to the opposite dome and superiorly to the root of the nose. The subperichondrial dissection over the dome can be continued medially between the two alar cartilages if required, incising the interdomal ligamentous attachments. The pointed ends of the scissors are brought back into the nasal cavity through the intercartilaginous and transfixion incisions (Fig. 14.7B).

Once the three incisions and the subperichondrial dissection of overlying soft tissues are completed, the alar cartilage is free, except at its medial and lateral ends. If it is not completely free, scissors are inserted into the marginal incision and the dissection is completed until the subperichondrial pocket extends from the marginal to the inter-cartilaginous/transfixion incision. The intercartilaginous incision should be long enough to permit adequate mobilization of the lateral crus for exposure. This dissection creates a bipedicled flap of alar cartilage lined with vestibular skin based medially and laterally. The alar cartilages are then "delivered" from the nostrils, similar to the handle of a bucket, by retraction with skin hooks, exposing the superficial surface of the cartilage (see Fig. 14.8).

➤ **STEP 3.** Exposure of the Nasal Dorsum and Root

Access to the nasal dorsum and root is gained through the intercartilaginous incision. Once the incision has been made through mucosa, submucosa, aponeurotic tissue, and perichondrium, sharp subperichondrial dissection with a scalpel or blunt dissection with sharp scissors

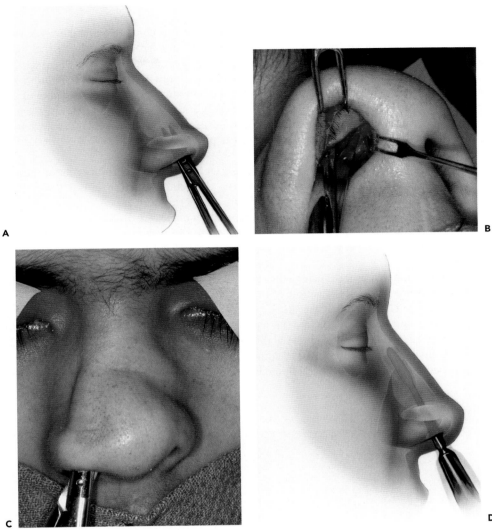

FIGURE 14.9 Scissor dissection over the upper nasal skeleton. Illustration **(A)** and photograph **(B)** showing insertion of the scissors through the intercartilaginous incision, superficial to the upper lateral cartilage. The scissors are advanced using a spreading motion until as much of the external nasal soft tissues as necessary for the surgical procedure has been dissected **(C)**. **D:** Illustration showing the use of a sharp periosteal elevator to dissect the nasal bones.

frees the soft tissues from the upper lateral cartilages (see Fig. 14.9). The dissection should be within the subperichondrial plane to prevent injury to the overlying musculature and blood vessels of the nose. Dissection to the inferior border of the nasal bones and across the midline to the opposite side is performed through a unilateral intercartilaginous incision. Retraction of the freed soft tissues allows a sharp incision to be made with a scalpel through the periosteum at the inferior edge of the nasal bones. Sharp periosteal elevators such as Cottle, Joseph, or Freer are useful for subperiosteal dissection of the nasal bones to the level that is necessary for the surgical procedure (Fig. 14.9D).

➤ **STEP 4.** Exposure of the Septum

The septal mucosa is stripped from the septal cartilage through the transfixion incision, using periosteal elevators. The mucoperichondrium is attached intimately to the septal cartilage, especially anteriorly, and is often difficult to separate initially (see Fig. 14.10). It may be necessary to begin by performing a sharp dissection with a scalpel. The blue–white appearance of the septal cartilage indicates that the operator is in the proper plane of dissection. Once the mucosa has been freed from the anterior septum, a Freer elevator is used in a sweeping motion to dissect the mucoperichondrium off the entire septal cartilage from the vomer to the dorsum and posteriorly over the perpendicular plate of the ethmoid (see Fig. 14.11).

The septal mucosa strips readily in most areas except along the inferior border of the septal cartilage, particularly anteriorly, where there is a grooved articulation with the vomer and premaxillary crest. In this area, the perichondrium and periosteum are continuous from side to side, and each fuse in the midline so that the dissection planes are discontinuous and form a barrier to elevation. This situation is further complicated by the common occurrence of spurs and deviations in this area. Attempts to forcibly elevate the lining may lead to tears in the mucosa.

The bidirectional approach, using superior and inferior "tunnels," allows isolation of this area and exposure for sharp elevation of the fused membranes on one side of the septum. The superior tunnel is created by elevating the mucoperichondrium and periosteum from the septal cartilage and ethmoid to where the septum meets the nasal crest of the maxilla and/or vomer (Fig. 14.11). The inferior tunnel is then created by dissecting submucosally down the transfixion incision to the anterior nasal spine and across the pyriform aperture. Extension of the transfixion incision onto the nasal floor facilitates the dissection and helps prevent mucosal

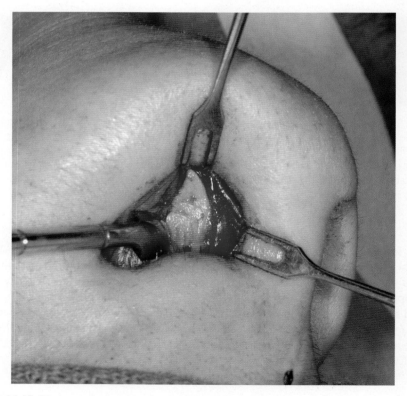

FIGURE 14.10 Photograph showing dissection of the nasal septal mucosa from the anterior septal angle using a Cottle elevator.

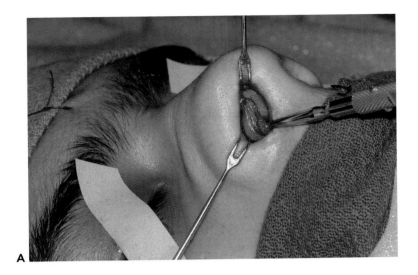

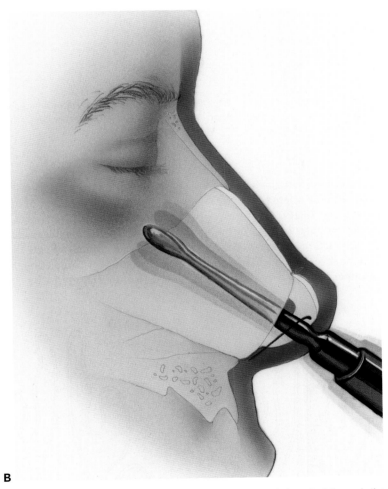

FIGURE 14.11 Submucosal elevation of the septum. The elevator is inserted through the transfixion incision **(A)** and mucosa is released to the level of the vomer/septal crest junction with the cartilaginous septum **(B)**.

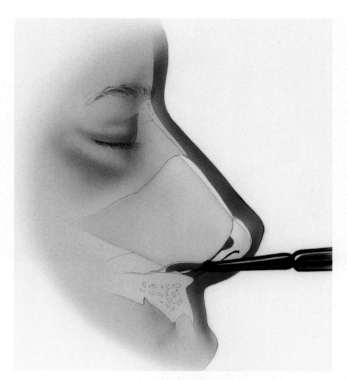

FIGURE 14.12 Submucosal elevation of the floor of the nose. The elevator is inserted through the transfixion incision and mucosa of the floor and septum is released to the level of the vomer/septal crest junction of the cartilaginous septum.

tearing. The mucoperiosteum is elevated off the nasal floor and up the nasal crest of the maxilla and vomer to the point where the septal mucosa is bound to the junction of the septum and these bones (see Fig. 14.12). The result is two submucosal tunnels, separated by submucosal adherence to the inferior edge of the septal cartilage and the maxillary crest/vomer (see Fig. 14.13A). Retraction of the mucosa from within these tunnels allows the submucosal attachments to be severed with sharp scissors or a scalpel, thereby completing the elevation of the entire mucoperichondrial–periosteal flap from the septum (Fig. 14.13B).

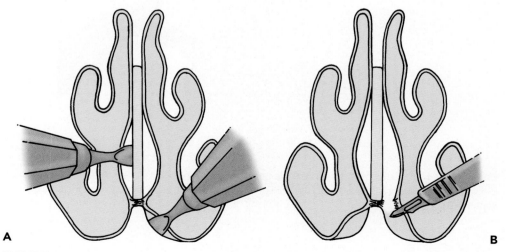

FIGURE 14.13 Submucosal dissection of the septum above and below the areas of adherence **(A)**, followed by incision through the adherent areas **(B)**.

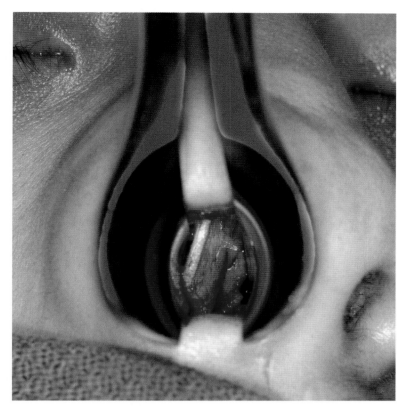

FIGURE 14.14 Photograph showing a deviated nasal septum that has been completely exposed by hemitransfixion and intercartilaginous incisions.

One can also dissect the mucoperichondrium off the opposite side of the nasal septum if necessary through either a hemitransfixion or a complete transfixion incision, exposing the entire nasal septum (see Fig. 14.14).

Mucosa on the undersurface of the upper lateral cartilage is also dissected through the combined intercartilaginous/transfixion incision to prevent its damage during resection procedures involving the nasal dorsum. A simple method to free the mucosa at the junction of the septum and upper lateral cartilage is to position a Freer elevator submucosally along the nasal septum just under the nasal dorsum and rotate the superior edge of the Freer elevator laterally. This maneuver separates the mucoperiosteum/mucoperichondrium from the undersurface of the nasal vault.

➤ STEP 5. Closure and Splints

All intranasal incisions are closed with resorbable suture, such as the 5-0 chromic catgut suture. If the septal mucosa was detached, placement of intranasal splints or packs will maintain mucosal approximation and help prevent hematoma formation during the healing process. Alternatively, trans-septal quilting sutures are useful in readapting the mucosa.

If the soft tissues of the nasal dorsum and tip have been elevated, an external nasal dressing may be applied to readapt the tissues to the underlying skeleton. After applying a thin coating of tincture of benzoin or other skin preparation solution over the skin of the nose and adjoining area, a paper tape is applied in overlapping layers from the root to the supratip area. A V-notch is cut out of a strip of tape to form a sling for tip support. An external nasal dressing is then applied.

INDEX

Note: Page numbers followed by "*f*" indicate figures.

A

Alar bases, resetting, 118
Alar cartilage delivery approach, 234–240
　intercartilaginous incision (limen vestibuli incision), 237–238, 237*f*, 238*f*
　marginal incision, 235–237, 236*f*
　subperichondrial dissection, 239–240, 239*f*, 240*f*
　transfixion incision, 237*f*, 238–239
Alar (lower lateral) cartilages, 216*f*, 217
Alar cinch suture, 118, 119*f*, 126, 134
Anterior maxilla and/or orbit, subperiosteal dissection of, 26–29
　inferior oblique muscle, 26–29, 29*f*
　inferior orbital fissure, 29, 29*f*
　infraorbital rim, 26, 27*f*–28*f*
　orbital floor and wall exposure, 29, 29*f*
Anterior septal angle, 218, 231*f*
Artery
　ethmoidal, 98, 100
　facial, 137–138, 139*f*, 154*f*, 155, 158, 158*f*, 159*f*
Atkinson, M. E., 153
Auriculotemporal nerve, 193–194

B

Bauer retractors, 147, 148*f*
Blepharoplasty incisions, 17, 70, 71*f*
Buccal fat pad, 82*f*, 84, 113–114, 114*f*, 140–142

C

Canthal tendons
　lateral
　　surgical anatomy of, 14–15, 14*f*, 15*f*
　　transconjunctival approaches, 46, 54–55
　medial
　　coronal approach, 98, 99*f*, 100, 101*f*
　　midfacial degloving approach, 121
　　surgical anatomy of, 15–16, 15*f*, 16*f*
　　transcaruncular approach, 55, 56
Cantholysis, 45, 46*f*
Canthopexy, lateral, 104
Canthotomy, lateral, 45, 54
Capsulopalpebral fascia, 43
Cornua (horns), levator aponeurosis, 68
Coronal approach, 81–106
　advantages, 81
　alternate incisions, 105–106

　postauricular placement, 105*f*
　zigzag incision, 106, 106*f*
closure, 104–105
　flat drain, use of, 104
　lateral canthopexy, 104
　periosteum, 104
　preauricular component, 105
　scalp incision, 105
　suture resuspension of soft tissues, 104
　temporalis fascia, oversuspension of, 104
　temporalis muscle, suspension of, 104
coronal flap, elevation of, 90–95
　bleeding, control of, 90–91
　flap dissection, 91, 92*f*
　pericranial flap, development of, 93
　periosteal incisions, 91–93
cranial bone grafts, harvesting, 103
exposure obtained, 87, 100, 101*f*
facial nerve, temporal branches of, 84–85, 86*f*
hemostatic techniques, 89
incision, 89–90
　below superior temporal line, 90, 91*f*
　crosshatching, 89, 90*f*
　initial, 89–90
　preauricular extension, 90
incision placement and preparation, 87–89, 89*f*
　hair, confining and gathering, 89, 89*f*
　hairline of patient, 87–89
　inferior access required, 88
　shaving of the head, 89
mandibular condyle/ramus, exposure of, 102
medial orbit, 85–87
　anterior one third of wall, 85
　bones of, 85
　middle one third of wall, 86
　posterior one third of wall, 86
periorbital areas, subperiosteal exposure of, 95–101
　ethmoidal artery, 98, 100
　lateral orbit, 98
　medial canthal tendons, 98, 99*f*, 100, 101*f*
　nasofrontal region, 98, 99*f*
　superior and medial orbital walls, 98
　supraorbital neurovascular bundle, release of, 95, 98*f*
scalp, layers of, 81–83
　galea, 81
　musculoaponeurotic layer, 81, 82*f*
　pericranium (periosteum), 82*f*, 83

　SCALP acronym, 81
　skin, 81, 82*f*
　subcutaneous tissue, 81, 82*f*
　subgaleal fascia, 81–83
　superficial musculoaponeurotic system, 81
　temporoparietal fascia, 81
temporal fossa, exposure of, 102
temporomandibular joint, exposure of, 102
temporoparietal region, layers of, 82*f*, 83–84
　buccal fat pad, 82*f*, 84
　subgaleal fascia, 83
　superficial temporal fat pad, 83*f*, 84
　temporalis fascia, 82*f*, 83, 83*f*
　temporalis muscle, 82*f*, 83, 83*f*
　temporoparietal fascia, 81, 82*f*, 83, 83*f*
zygomatic arch, exposure of, 93–95, 97*f*
Cottle elevator, 125, 226, 231*f*, 241, 242*f*
Cranial bone graft harvest, 103

D

Dingman, R. L., 153

E

Endonasal approach, 234–245
　alar cartilage delivery approach (*see* Alar cartilage delivery approach)
　closure and splints, 245
　nasal dorsum and root, exposure of, 240–241
　preparation, 234
　septum, exposure of, 242–245
　vasoconstriction, 234
Ethmoidal artery, 98, 100
External (open) approach, 215–233
　closure, 226
　external nasal bony framework, 215, 216*f*
　external nasal cartilage framework, 215–218
　　alar (lower lateral) cartilages, 216*f*, 217
　　sesamoids, 215, 216*f*
　　upper lateral (triangular) cartilages, 215, 216*f*
　external skeletonization of the nose, 224–226
　　alar cartilages, dissection of, 226, 227*f*
　　external nose, exposure of, 226, 229*f*
　　lower lateral cartilages, dissection of, 224–226

External (open) approach (*Continued*)
  medial crura, subperichondrial
    dissection of, 224
  nasal dorsum, dissection of, 226, 228*f*
  marginal and transcolumellar incisions,
    221, 221*f*–224*f*
  nasal septum, 218, 219*f*
  nasal soft tissues, 218
  preparation, 219
  scroll area, 215, 217*f*
  septum, exposure of, 226, 230*f*–231*f*
  splints, 226, 233*f*
  vasoconstriction, 219, 220*f*

F

Facial artery, 137–138, 139*f*, 154*f*, 155, 158,
  158*f*, 159*f*
Facial nerve
  branching pattern of, 169–170, 171*f*,
    172, 173
  marginal mandibular branches, 153, 160,
    170, 173–176
  temporal branches, 84–85, 86*f*, 194, 195*f*
Facial skeletal surgery. *See also specific*
    approaches
  incision placement, 3–5
    age, 3
    anatomic features, 3–4
    cosmetic considerations, 3
    facial expression, muscles and nerves
      of, 3
    favorable sites, 5
    length of incision, 4
    lines of minimal tension (relaxed skin
      tension lines), 4–5
    neurovascular structures, 4
    patient expectations, 4
    perpendicular, 4
    sensory nerves, 3
Facial vein, 138, 139*f*, 154*f*, 155, 158, 158*f*,
  159*f*
Fascia
  capsulopalpebral, 43
  parotideomasseteric, 193
  subgaleal, 81–83
  temporalis, 82*f*, 83, 83*f*, 91
  temporoparietal, 81, 82*f*, 83
Freer elevator, 20*f*, 59, 117, 125, 226, 241,
  242, 245

G

Galea, 81
Grabb, W. C., 153
Great auricular nerve, 185, 186*f*

H

Hinds, E. C., 171
Horner muscle, 55–57, 59, 60

I

Inferior fornix incision, 41
Infraciliary incision. *See* Subciliary incision
Infraorbital groove, 16

Infraorbital nerve, 128, 129*f*
Infraorbital neurovascular bundle, 16, 116,
  117
Intercartilaginous incision, 122–123
Intranasal incisions, 122–124
  circumvestibularity, ensuring, 124, 125*f*
  intercartilaginous incision (limen
    vestibuli incision), 122–123
  piriform aperture, 122*f*, 123
  transfixion incision, 122*f*, 123, 124*f*
Ipsilateral lip drooping, 128

J

Jaeger Lid Plate, 48*f*, 59
Joseph elevator, 125

L

Lacrimal canaliculi, 15
Lacrimal crest, 15–16
Lacrimal puncta, 15
Lacrimal sac, 15
Lacrimal sac fossa, 55
Lateral canthal tendons. *See* Canthal
    tendons
LaVasseur-Merrill retractor, 147
Le Fort osteotomies, 126
Levator anguli oris, 112
Levator aponeurosis, 68, 69*f*, 72*f*
Levator labii superioris, 112, 128, 129*f*
Levator labii superioris alaeque nasi, 112
Limen vestibuli incision, 122–123
Lines of minimal tension, 4–5
Loose areolar layer, 81–83
Lower eyelid approaches, 10–40
  exposure obtained, 9
  extended incisions, 37–40
  lower eyelid anatomy, 10–14, 42, 43*f*
    capsulopalpebral fascia, 43
    infraorbital groove, 16
    lateral canthal tendon, 14–15, 14*f*, 15*f*
    lower eyelid retractors, 42–43, 43*f*
    medial canthal tendon, 15–16,
      15*f*, 16*f*
    Meibomian glands, 14
    orbicularis oculi muscle, 10–14
    orbital septum, 10*f*, 12–14, 13*f*
    palpebral conjunctiva, 10*f*, 14
    skin, 11
    tarsus/tarsal plate, 10*f*, 12–14
  poor cosmetic results, 9*f*
  subciliary approach, 17–32
    anterior maxilla and/or orbit,
      subperiosteal dissection of, 26–29
    closure, 30, 31*f*
    incision placement, 16, 20*f*
    lower-eyelid suspensory suture, 30, 32*f*
    periosteal incision, 26, 26*f*
    pretarsal and preseptal portions,
      incision between, 24, 25*f*
    scleral shell, use of, 18
    skin flap dissection, 17
    skin incision, 21
    skin-muscle flap dissection, 17
    step dissection, 17
    subcutaneous dissection, 21, 21*f*, 22*f*

suborbicularis dissection, 23, 23*f*, 24*f*
    temporary tarsorrhaphy, 18, 18*f*, 19*f*, 21*f*
  subtarsal approach, 32–36
    advantages, 32
    incision placement, 32–33
    relaxed skin tension lines, 32–33
    skin incision, 33, 34*f*
    suborbicularis dissection, 33, 35*f*–36*f*

M

Mandibular ramus
  coronal approach exposure, 102
  subperiosteal dissection, 145–147
Mandibular vestibular approach, 137–150
  advantages, 137
  buccal fat pad, 140–141
  closure, 147–150
    mentalis muscle, suturing, 147–150
    posterior to anterior regions, 147, 149*f*
    suspension dressing, placement of, 149
  complications, 137
  facial artery, 137–138, 139*f*
  facial vein, 138, 139*f*
  incision, 141–145
    buccal fat pad, preventing herniation
      of, 142
    edentulous mandible, 142
    mandible, body and posterior portion,
      142
    mentalis muscle, 141–142
    mental nerve, avoiding, 142, 145
    mucosa, anterior region of lip, 141
  mandible, subperiosteal dissection of,
    145–147
    Bauer retractors, 147, 148*f*
    masseter muscle, 147
    mentalis muscle, stripping, 145, 145*f*
    mental nerves, 145
    notched right-angle retractors, 145, 147*f*
    ramus, 145–147, 147*f*
  mentalis muscle, 138–140
  mental nerve, 137, 138*f*
  vasoconstriction, 141
Maxillary vestibular approach, 111–121
  advantages, 111
  anterior maxilla and zygoma,
    subperiosteal dissection of, 116–117
  buccal fat pad, 113, 114*f*
  closure, 118–121
    alar base, identification and resetting
      of, 118
    horizontal incision, 120
    V-Y closure, vestibular incision, 118–121
  exposure obtained, 114, 118, 118*f*
  incision placement, 115–116
  infraorbital nerve, 111
  nasal cavity, submucosal dissection of,
    117–118
  nasolabial musculature, 112–113
    effects of surgery on, 113*f*
    levator anguli oris, 112
    levator labii superioris, 112
    levator labii superioris alaeque nasi, 112
    nasalis group, 112
    orbicularis oris, 112
  vasoconstriction, 115

Medial canthal tendons. *See* Canthal tendons
Medial orbit, 85–87, 98–100. *See also* Transconjunctival approaches
Meibomian glands, 14
Mentalis muscle, 138–140, 145, 145*f*
Mental nerves, 137, 138*f*, 145
Midfacial degloving approach, 121–127. *See also* Maxillary vestibular approach
  advantages, 121
  exposure obtained, 127*f*
  technique, 121–127
    anesthesia, 121
    closure, 126
    intranasal incisions, 122–124
    maxillary vestibular incision, 125–126
    midfacial osteotomies, 126
    nasal dorsum and root, exposure of, 124–125
    nose, preparation of, 121–122
    subperiosteal exposure, 125–126
    vasoconstriction, 121–122
Midfacial osteotomies, 126
Modified Blair incision, 183, 184*f*
Müller muscle/tarsus complex, 68–70
Musculoaponeurotic layer, 81, 82*f*

N

Nasal bones, 218, 219*f*
Nasalis group, 112
Nasal septum, 218
Nasal skeleton, approaches to. *See* External (open) approach
Nasal soft tissues, 218
Nasolabial musculature. *See under* Maxillary vestibular approach
Nerve(s)
  auriculotemporal, 193–194
  facial
    branching pattern of, 169–170, 171*f*, 172, 173
    marginal mandibular branches, 153, 160, 170, 173–176
    temporal branches, 84–85, 86*f*, 194, 195*f*
  great auricular, 185, 186f
  infraorbital, 128, 129f
  mental, 137, 138f, 145
  sensory, 3
  zygomatico-facial, 128
  zygomatico-frontal, 128
Node of Stahr, 160
Nose, surgical anatomy of, 215–217, 221
  external nasal bony framework, 215, 216*f*
  external nasal cartilage framework, 215–217
    alar (lower lateral) cartilages, 216*f*, 217
    sesamoids, 215, 216*f*
    upper lateral (triangular) cartilages, 215, 216*f*
  nasal septum, 218
  nasal soft tissues, 218
  scroll area, 215, 217*f*
  soft triangle, 221
Notched right-angle retractors, 145, 147*f*

O

Orbicularis oculi muscle, 10–14, 55, 68, 69*f*, 71, 72*f*, 73*f*
  innervation and blood supply, 12
  orbital portion, 11
  palpebral portion, 11–12
  preseptal portion, 11
  pretarsal portion, 11, 12*f*
Orbicularis oris, 112, 128, 129*f*
Orbital septum/levator aponeurosis complex, 68
Orbital septum/tarsus, 10*f*, 12–14, 13*f*
Osteotomies, midfacial, 126

P

Palpebral conjunctiva, 10*f*, 14
Paralyzed face, 3
Parotideomasseteric fascia, 193
Parotid gland, 193
Pars lacrimalis. *See* Horner muscle
Pericranium (periosteum), 82*f*, 83
Piriform aperture, 116–118, 122*f*, 123
Platysma muscle, 156, 157*f*, 172, 173*f*
Preauricular approach
  auriculotemporal nerve, 193–194
  extended incisions, 211
    endaural incision (retrotragal), 211, 212*f*
    oblique anterosuperior extension (hockey stick), 211
    retroauricular skin incision, 211, 212*f*
  parotideomasseteric fascia, 193
  parotid gland, 193
  superficial temporal vessels, 193, 194*f*
  technique, 198–211
    closure, 209, 210*f*
    incision placement, 198
    interarticular spaces, exposing, 205–208
    preparation and draping, 198
    skin incision, 199, 199*f*
    temporal branches, protection of, 194–195
    temporomandibular joint capsule, dissection to, 199–205
    vasoconstriction, 198
  temporal branches, facial nerve, 194, 195*f*
  temporomandibular joint, 195–197
    articular capsule, 195–197
    articular disk, 195–196
    capsule, 195, 196*f*
  temporoparietal region, layers of, 197–198
    subgaleal fascia, 197
    superficial temporal fat pad, 198
    temporalis fascia, 198
    temporoparietal fascia, 197
Pterygomasseteric sling, 158–160, 173–178

R

Raney clips, 90
Relaxed skin tension lines, 4–5, 32, 33*f*

Retromandibular approach, 169–184
  closure, 181–183
  combining approaches, 183
  facial nerve, 169–170, 170*f*, 171*f*
    branching pattern of, 169–170, 171*f*
    marginal mandibular branch, 170
  modified Blair incision, 183, 184*f*
  preparation and draping, 171
  pterygomasseteric sling, dissection to, 173–176
    facial nerve branches, identifying with nerve stimulator, 173
    marginal mandibular branch, retracting, 173–176
    parotid gland, dissection through, 173, 173*f*
    platysma muscle, superficial musculoaponeurotic system, and parotid capsule fusion, incising through, 173, 173f
    retromandibular vein, 174–175*f*, 176
  pterygomasseteric sling, division of, 176–178
  retromandibular vein, 170–171, 171*f*
  sigmoid notch retractor, use of, 178
  skin incision, 171, 173
  submasseteric dissection, 178–180
    gonial angle region, screw and traction wire application to, 180
    masseter muscle, stripping and retraction of, 178, 179*f*
  vasoconstriction, 172
Retromandibular vein, 174–175*f*, 176
Rhytidectomy approach
  advantages and disadvantages, 185
  great auricular nerve, 185, 186*f*
  technique, 185–189
    closure, 189, 189*f*
    incision placement, 185–187
    preparation and draping, 185
    retromandibular approach, 188, 188*f*
    skin flap elevation and dissection, 187–188
    skin incision, 187
    vasoconstriction, 185–187

S

Scalp, layers of. *See under* Coronal approach
Scroll area, 215, 217*f*
Semilunar fold (plica semilunaris), 56, 57*f*, 58*f*
Sesamoids, 215, 216*f*
Sigmoid notch retractors, 163, 163*f*, 178
Skin crease approach. *See* Subtarsal approach
SMAS. *See* Superficial musculoaponeurotic system (SMAS)
Soft triangle, 221
Split-thickness skin graft, 133, 133*f*
Stevens scissors, 59
Subaponeurotic plane, 81–83
Subciliary incision, 17. *See also* Lower eyelid approaches
Subgaleal fascia, 81–83, 197

Submandibular approach, 153–168
  closure, 164, 164f
  extended incisions
    complete bilateral exposure, 168, 168f
    increased ipsilateral exposure, 165–166f
    lower lip, surgical splitting of, 165–168, 167f
  facial artery, 154f, 155
  facial vein, 154f, 155
  incision placement, 153, 155
    inferior border of mandible, 153, 155
    mandibular fractures, 155
    resting skin tension lines, 156f
  marginal mandibular branch, facial nerve, 153
  platysma muscle, incising, 156, 157f
  preparation and draping, 155
  pterygomasseteric muscular sling, dissection to, 158–160
    electrical nerve stimulator, use of, 160
    facial vein and artery, 158, 158f, 159f
    fascia, dissection through, 158–160
    marginal mandibular branch, facial nerve, 160
    Node of Stahr, 160
    submandibular salivary gland, retraction of, 160
  pterygomasseteric sling, division of, 160–163
  skin incision, 156
  submasseteric dissection, 162, 163f
  vasoconstriction, 155
Subtarsal approach, 32–36. See under Lower eyelid approaches
  advantages, 32
  incision placement, 32–33
  relaxed skin tension lines, 32–33
  skin incision, 33, 34f
  suborbicularis dissection, 33, 35f–36f
Superficial musculoaponeurotic system (SMAS), 81, 173, 173f, 197
Superficial temporal fascia, 197
Superficial temporal fat pad, 83f, 84, 96f, 198
Superficial temporal vessels, 193, 194f
Supraorbital eyebrow approach, 65–67
  advantages and disadvantages, 65
  limited access and exposure, 65, 67f
  technique, 65–67
    closure, 67
    periosteal incision, 66
    skin incision, 65–66
    subperiosteal dissection (lateral orbital rim/lateral orbit), 67
    vasoconstriction, 65
Supratarsal fold approach. See Upper eyelid approach
Suprazygomatic superficial musculoaponeurotic system, 197

T

Tarsal glands, 14
Tarsal plate
  conjunctiva, incision of, 47, 47f
  lower eyelid, 10f, 12–14

upper eyelid, 68, 69
Tarsorrhaphy suture
  subciliary approach, 17–32
  upper eyelid approach, 70
Temporal hollowing, 94
Temporalis fascia, 82f, 83, 83f, 91, 198
Temporalis muscle, 82f, 83, 104
Temporomandibular joint (TMJ)
  articular capsule, 195–197
  articular disk, 195–196
  capsule, 195, 196f
  coronal approach exposure, 102
  retroauricular approach, 211, 212f
Temporoparietal fascia, 81, 82f, 83, 197
Temporoparietal region layers. See Coronal approach; Preauricular approach
Thermoplastic splint, to external nose, 226, 233f
TMJ. See Temporomandibular joint (TMJ)
Transcaruncular approach. See Transconjunctival approaches
Transconjunctival approaches, 41–64
  combining, 61–64
  extended (frontozygomatic area exposure), 54–55
  traditional incision (inferior fornix incision), 41–54
    cantholysis, 45, 46f
    closure, 50–54
    corneal shield placement, 44, 47, 48f
    lateral canthotomy, 45
    lower eyelid anatomy, 42, 43f
    periosteal incision, 49
    preseptal and retroseptal approaches, 41, 42f
    subperiosteal orbital dissection, 49
    traction sutures, lower eyelid, 44, 45
    transconjunctival incision, 46–49
    vasoconstriction, 43, 44f
  transcaruncular (medial orbit), 58–61
    caruncle, 56–58
    closure, 60
    Horner muscle (pars lacrimalis), 55–57, 59, 60
    lacrimal sac fossa, 55
    medial canthal tendon, 55
    orbicularis oculi muscle, 55
    periosteal incision and exposure, 60, 60f, 61f
    semilunar fold (plica semilunaris), 56, 57f, 58f
    subconjunctival dissection, 59–60
    transconjunctival incision, 59
    vasoconstriction, 58
Transfixion incision, 122f, 123, 124f
Trans-septal quilting sutures, 226
Triangular cartilages, 215, 216f

U

Upper blepharoplasty approach. See Upper eyelid approach
Upper eyelid approach, 68–78
  technique, 70–78
    blepharoplasty incisions, 70, 71f
    closure, 73, 76f, 77f, 78f

corneal protection, 70
    incision positioning and marking, 70
    periosteal incision, 73
    skin incision, 71
    skin-muscle flap, undermining of, 73, 73f
    subperiosteal dissection (lateral orbital rim/lateral orbit), 73, 74f, 75f
    vasoconstriction, 71, 71f
  upper eyelid anatomy, 68–70
    cornua (horns), 68
    five layers of, 68, 69f
    Müller muscle/tarsus complex, 68–70
    orbital septum/levator aponeurosis complex, 68
    tarsal plate, 68–70

V

V-Y closure, vestibular incision, 118–121, 126

W

Weber-Fergusson approach, 109, 128–136
  closure, 133–136
    intraoral, 134
    resuspension of cheek flap, 134f
    skin and upper lip, 134, 136f
    split-thickness skin graft, 133, 133f
    transnasal suturing (alar cinch), 134
  exposure obtained, 133f
  flap dissection from maxilla, 131–133, 132f, 133f
    infraorbital neurovascular bundle, 132
    supraperiosteal dissection, 131
  incision, 128–131
    edentulous spaces, 131
    intraoral, 130f, 131
    lateral nasal, 130
    lip, 128–130
    lower eyelid extension, 130–131, 130f
    subnasal, 130
    upper eyelid extension, 130
  lateral orbital area, 128
    infraorbital nerve, 128, 129f
    zygomatico-facial nerve, 128
    zygomatico-frontal nerve, 128
  lip, anatomy of, 128, 129f
    levator labii superioris, 128
    orbicularis oris, 128
  vasoconstriction, 128
Westcott scissors, 59

Z

Zariah, H. A., 153
Zigzag incision, 106, 106f
Zygoma, 117
Zygomatic arch
  coronal approach exposure, 93–95, 97f
  maxillary vestibular approach exposure, 117
Zygomatico-facial nerve, 128
Zygomatico-frontal nerve, 128
Zygomaticomaxillary buttress, 116–117